NEUROPUNCTURE®
CUTTING EDGE NEUROSCIENCE ACUPUNCTURE SYSTEM™

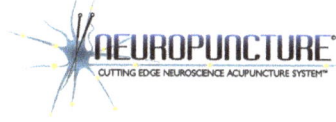

NEUROPUNCTURE™ CASE STUDIES AND CLINICAL APPLICATIONS: VOLUME 1

By Dr. Michael D. Corradino and Dr. Helen K. Law

Published 2020 by Neuropuncture, Inc.

ISBN: 978-0-9893846-1-2

Cover design: AG Creative Solutions
Interior layout: AG Creative Solutions

Neuropuncture™ Case Studies and Clinical Applications: Volume 1 was written by Dr. Michael D. Corradino and Dr. Helen K. Law

For more information email info@neuropuncture.com

CONTENTS

FOREWORD

The foundations of Traditional Chinese Medicine (TCM) have been traced back to the third millennium BC, a time when disease was believed to be the result of demonic and spiritual forces. Between the fifth and third centuries BC, the *Huangdi Neijing*, the most important historical text on Chinese medicine, was composed, replacing such shamanistic beliefs with theories incorporating diet, environment, and age as factors contributing to health. It organized the framework of yin and yang and qi and the five elements and continues to prove influential as a reference work for practitioners of TCM well into the modern era (Curan 2008). Today, the practice has greatly expanded and is used by a quarter of the world's population across the globe, with more than ten million acupuncture treatments administered annually in the United States alone. Its rise in popularity, particularly in the West, can be attributed in part to its effectiveness for pain relief and in part to a rapidly increasing body of scientific research that supports its efficacy (Hao and Mittelman 2014).

Having been raised in a family of highly respected traditional Chinese medicine physicians in Hong Kong, acupuncture has always been a large part of my life. However, I did not initially follow in their footsteps. I took a detour and studied aerospace engineering and computer science, leading to a long career in aerospace research at Princeton University. But something was always calling me back, and I eventually responded to my calling as a doctor of Chinese medicine. In the twenty years since starting my acupuncture practice, it has become my passion, and I have never once looked back. It is a fascinating art and science in that the more you learn, the more you want to learn. I have studied many different methods and styles of acupuncture, approaching it conceptually from all angles. In the clinic, each method has shown its strengths, and the mastery of fluidly employing each when called for has led to a continuously expanding repertoire of conditions I have been able to successfully improve. However, I have never stopped asking the question: How do we explain all these different approaches with one theory?

Instinctually, I have always believed acupuncture to be a type of neuroscience. I even called myself an "Acupuncture Neurologist." But after years of following the research that linked acupuncture to neuroscience, I was still unable to find a systematic approach that clearly explained the neurophysiology mechanisms of acupuncture. That is, until I met Dr. Michael Corradino. I attended Dr. Corradino's first workshop in June of 2019 and immediately recognized it as the framework I had been searching for. Dr. Corradino presented a complete neuroscience acupuncture system he calls "Neuropuncture." He built largely on fifty years of research by Dr. Ji-sheng Han and Dr. Corradino's understandings and investigations into neuroscience and neurophysiology. Dr. Ji-sheng Han in 1940 began studying the connection between neuroscience and electrical acupuncture in the endorphin arena. The methodology of Neuropuncture combines the research of electrical acupuncture's effects on specific neural receptors by investigating Western medical sciences and integrating them with the holistic TCM framework. Furthermore, Dr. Corradino created the treatment prescriptions that are patent-pending, evidence-based, and clinically reproducible.

The one question my patients ask more than any other is this: How does acupuncture work? I would always answer the conventional way, explaining that qi or vital energy flows along the twelve meridians in the body. Blockages in this flow resulted in illness. Acupuncture worked by removing these blockages, hence creating the balance and harmony of energy within the body. While this model still has much to offer us, the terminology and conceptual framework does not align with that of twenty-first-century medical sciences and thus is easy to misinterpret within a different paradigm. Furthermore, collaboration with a patient's Western-medicine physicians is limited due to this incompatibility of language and ideas. Neuropuncture has removed many of these barriers, bridging the chasm that has, for so long, separated Eastern and Western medical thought.

In 2012, Dr. Corradino laid the foundation of Neuropuncture in his first book, *Neuropuncture: A Clinical Handbook of Neuroscience Acupuncture*. Dr. Corradino published his second edition of *Neuropuncture* in 2017 and has been involved in groundbreaking electrical acupuncture research since 2010. I now feel that it is time to present to the world the clinical impact Neuropuncture has provided to our practitioners and their patients worldwide. In this book, we build on the theory through examination of real case studies. The content includes the commonly seen clinical conditions. Case studies were clinically performed in various clinics all over the world, utilizing strictly Neuropuncture theory and prescriptions. The purpose of this book is to increase the understanding of students who are interested in learning this Neuropuncture system. Additionally, it is our hope that this book will also influence Western medical doctors and help to introduce this system to them in a language that they are familiar with and help to bridge the gap between these two medical systems in a seamless fashion.

Ever since incorporating the Neuropuncture system into my practice, I've found that it has not only become a treatment protocol I turn to on a daily basis, but it also sheds new light on every other technique I continue to employ. Within its neurophysiological framework, I am able to quickly identify the causes of my patients' complaints and devise treatment prescriptions that have shown remarkable results in record time. Many of these fascinating and complex cases and their resolutions are presented, in detail, in this book. Neuropuncture has added great value to my practice and sparked a fresh perspective that I am just beginning to explore more deeply and want to share with you. I believe Neuropuncture is leading the way to the future of acupuncture medicine, integrating the wisdom of the East with the science of the West.

Dr. Corradino's passion and enthusiasm are contagious; his knowledge, experience, and intuition are second to none. I am so fortunate to have had the opportunity to study with him, and I'm thrilled to collaborate with him in the writing of this book.

Helen Law
Princeton, New Jersey 2020

References

Curan, J., Locum, GP & Glasgow. 2008. "Review: The Yellow Emperor's Classic of Internal Medicine." *The BMJ* 336(7647) (April 5): 777. https://www.ncbi.nlm.nih.gov/pmc/articles/PMC2287209/.

Hao, J.J. and Mittelman, M. 2014. "Acupuncture: Past, Present, and Future." *Global Advances in Health and Medicine* 3, no. 4 (July).

Ulett, G.A., Han, S., & Han, JS. Electroacupuncture: Mechanisms and Clinical Application. *BIOL. PSYCHIATRY*. 1998,44:129-138.

ACKNOWLEDGMENTS

I would like to express my most heartfelt gratitude to Dr. Michael Corradino for giving me the opportunity to collaborate with him on the writing of *Neuropuncture Case Studies: Volume 1*. In working closely with him, I was able to dive deeply into the critical analysis of neuropathophysiology, forever changing my practice and my understanding of the human body. I also wish to thank all the Neuropuncture practitioners who shared their cases and experience. This collection is a testament of their generosity and community spirit.

Finally, none of this would have been possible without my family. Their encouragement and support throughout the COVID-19 pandemic allowed me to focus on this project. My special thanks to my son, Jeffrey Law, for our many discussions, which helped me organize my ideas.

Dr. Helen Law

It has been my absolute pleasure and honor to have worked with Dr. Helen Law on this collaboration, and I would like to sincerely thank her for her hard work, her family's sacrifice, and her vision on this project. She is truly an amazing person and a very special practitioner, and it fills my heart with emotion to see her commitment to Neuropuncture. After all, it was her idea for me to bring a book of Neuropuncture case studies to the world to illustrate Neuropuncture's clinical effectiveness and Neuropuncture's twenty-first-century medical applications. I also would like to extend a very special thank you to "mia Bambina, Ana" for all her patience, support, and hours of her time in the professional design work and layout of this book. I so very much appreciate you and your amazing talent, and I thank you for all your time, energy, and love in this project, once again.

Throughout this COVID-19 pandemic, we were able to use our time to compile and present these cases from my NeuroLab members around the world. So, I would also like to thank all of them for their dedication, understanding, commitment, and discipline in learning and applying Neuropuncture, the only complete neuroscience acupuncture system. It has been an incredible journey that began with a burning curiosity about neuroscience and acupuncture and continued with printing out and compiling research in binders, creating treatment prescriptions, then testing them with my amazing patients, and witnessing the astonishing clinical outcomes. The journey continued through repetition of the testing and observing the same astonishing clinical outcomes, gathering the data and writing it all down, and then sharing it and teaching it around the world, to now receiving these Neuropuncture clinical cases from those practitioners…and there is still so much more to come!

Dr. Michael Corradino

ABOUT THE AUTHORS

Helen Law, PhD, DAc, LAc

Dr. Helen Law graduated from Pacific College of Health and Science in 2000 with a Master of Acupuncture degree and in 2019 as a Doctor of Acupuncture. In 2007, she was a visiting scholar at Wenjing Hospital, China Academy of Chinese Medical Sciences in Beijing, where she specialized in orthopedics and traumatology. She is the director of Princeton Integrative Health, where acupuncturists, herbalists, medical doctors, naturopathic physicians, medical massage therapists, and craniosacral therapists all work together with one goal—to help patients rehabilitate their bodies back to states of health.

In over twenty years of practice in the field of integrative medicine, Dr. Law has worked closely with medical doctors in disciplines such as sports medicine, physiatry, neurology, pain management, gastroenterology, infertility, and rheumatology. For eight years, she worked at the Hospital for Special Surgery Integrative Care Center in New York where she integrated acupuncture with traditional medical procedures, bringing Western and Eastern philosophies closer together. Dr. Law has been named the Top Doctor in New Jersey for the past ten consecutive years and has been voted into the Hall of Fame of Best Doctors in Princeton.

It is the author's hope to reach as many Neuropuncture practitioners who are learning and practicing this amazing system as possible and share these incredible clinical outcomes with the medical profession at large. Acupuncturists and medical doctors who seek to learn about this amazing tool may also find this volume a useful treatise on the connection between acupuncture and neuroscience.

Michael Corradino, MSTOM, DAOM, AP

Dr. Michael Corradino has been studying traditional Chinese medicine and the science of acupuncture for the past thirty years. He has been in the field of integrated acupuncture and clinically practicing for the past twenty-five years. He has owned clinics on campuses of hospitals, has worked in integrated pain centers alongside medical doctors, and has been the director of integrated medicine for chemical dependency centers. He was in the first graduating class in the country to receive the Doctor of Acupuncture and Oriental Medicine. After traveling to China with the late Alex Tiberi in 2006, he began working on his first *Neuropuncture Workbook*.

Since then, Dr. Corradino has published two Neuropuncture clinical manuals (first and second editions), has published research, and has been involved in several neuroscience electroacupuncture research projects. He has traveled to China to further investigate AAA (acupuncture-assisted anesthesia) and has been flown around the world to teach Neuropuncture. Now this will be the third Neuropuncture book.

Dr. Corradino has been studying and clinically applying neuroscience acupuncture research throughout his professional career. He is a firm believer that we and our profession at large must embrace and apply twenty-first-century medical sciences to our medicine in order for it to thrive. He continues to be involved in groundbreaking electroacupuncture research to this date and is constantly improving his Neuropuncture system. Neuropuncture is his professional lifelong work, and he is proud to have had the courage to bring this to his profession and now witness the amazing impact it has had not only on the profession but also on practitioners and their patients worldwide. Dr. Corradino is excited to now offer Level One Clinical Neuropuncture certifications and Neuropuncture Instructor Certifications and will soon offer an internationally accredited OMD-Neuropuncture degree.

MEDICAL DISCLAIMER

Neuropuncture Inc. does not recommend, endorse, or make any representation about the efficacy, appropriateness, or suitability of any specific tests, products, procedures, treatments, services, opinions, health-care providers, or other information that may be contained in or available throughout this book. NEUROPUNCTURE, INC., IS NOT RESPONSIBLE NOR LIABLE FOR ANY ADVICE, COURSE OF TREATMENT, OR DIAGNOSIS OR ANY OTHER INFORMATION, SERVICES, OR PRODUCTS THAT YOU OBTAIN THROUGH THIS BOOK. With the following Neuropuncture Prescriptions (Rxs) that have been presented, it is important to understand that each case has to be individually evaluated and treated accordingly, and slight modifications of Rxs sometimes are needed. For correct Neuropuncture training, please contact Dr. Corradino.

INTRODUCTION

Neuropuncture is the only complete neuroscience acupuncture system in the world that has been created by a traditionally trained acupuncturist *for* the traditionally trained acupuncturist *and* anyone else who wants to learn how to apply twenty-first-century medical sciences to the classical acupuncture model, in an effort to bring acupuncture into the heart of mainstream medicine as opposed to leaving it on the outskirts. A "complete neuroscience acupuncture system" refers to the broad clinical application that Neuropuncture offers to any and all medical cases with which licensed acupuncturists are presented—from mental health conditions and internal medical conditions to orthopedic and pain management, including body, auricular, and scalp neuroscience acupuncture systems.

The human nervous system permeates and communicates with every cell and organ system on every level. Therefore, when individuals learn Neuropuncture's principles, they learn how to neuro-modulate, neuro-regulate, and neuro-rehabilitate the nervous system back into homeostasis and return the patient back to health. In Neuropuncture, we believe that our very unique, powerful neural networks are the often-mistranslated classical Chinese medical terms of *Mai* 脉 and *Jing luo* 经络. We believe that these neural network pathways have been miscommunicated as meridians or energy channels for too many decades. We also see the neuroscience evidence clearly in the classical *Deqi* 得气 phenomena represented below. The fact that our ancient predecessors acknowledged the *Deqi* 得气 sensation illustrates that they were stimulating the nervous system and that those transmissions terminated in the brain, our master organic CPU, which controls every aspect and function in the human body.

Table I - De Qi sensations and nerve association

Classical DeQi Sensation	Neural Fiber Association
Heaviness	A-delta, III muscle fiber
Soreness	C-fiber
Numbness	A-gamma
Vibration ("ants crawling on the skin")	A-beta
Achy ("deep muscle ache")	IV muscle fiber
Cold	A-delta
Hot	C-fiber, IV muscle fiber
Pinprick ("slight pain")	A-delta, C-fiber

The Neuropuncture Trinity, also referred to as the Neuropuncture Foundations, is the fundamental framework of neuroscience knowledge that empowers the practitioner to apply twenty-first-century medical sciences to our classical Traditional Chinese Medicine (TCM) acupuncture model. It has three sections, hence the term *trinity*. Each section is supported with evidence-based neuroanatomy, published medical research, and electrical sciences and has been clinically proven by the creator and licensed practitioners around the world. This also empowers the practitioner with the language to best communicate exactly how and what we are performing and what we expect our clinical outcomes to be.

The first section describes the Neuropuncture Neurophysiological Mechanisms, and these, when fully understood, will explain all and any clinical phenomena of any acupuncture technique or system. The second section, which covers the Neuropuncture Treatment Principles, teaches the practitioner how to apply the neurophysiological mechanisms to any medical case or medical diagnosis. By identifying the root underlying neuropathology of the condition, the Neuropuncture Treatment Principles help focus the treatment to target and heal the nervous tissue. The third section is on the Neuropuncture Electrical Techniques. It is understood in Neuropuncture, and is supported by published research, that electroacupuncture (EA) is superior than manual acupuncture, especially in the treatment of pain and in creating reproducible clinical outcomes. So, we must understand the electrical sciences and how to safely apply those sciences to neuro-modulate, neuro-regulate, and neuro-rehabilitate the nervous system properly.

When a trained practitioner understands the Neuropuncture Trinity and learns how to utilize it, the practitioner has the tools to create three special items that are specific to the Neuropuncture system: a Neuropuncture Rx (a functional acupuncture point/ unit prescription), a Neuropuncture dosage (the electrical parameters/electrical signature), and a Neuropuncture treatment plan (based on gene expression and neuroplasticity principles). In the Neuropuncture system, we always maintain the classical TCM holistic approach to healing our patient's entire system, utilizing other modalities to correct behavior, lifestyles, diet, and mind/body balance—but we understand that acupuncture is neuroscience and therefore apply those strategies while still using liniments, moxa, cupping, TDP (infrared heat lamp), laser, AIT (acupuncture injection therapy), traditional Tui Na, herbal medicine, dietary adjustments, nutraceuticals, and more.

Table II - Neuropuncture mechanisms and treatment principles

Neuropuncture neurophysiological mechanisms	Neuropuncture treatment principles
1. Local effect	1. Harness local effect
2. Spinal segmental	2. Target specific nerve
3. Endogenous Opioid Circuit (EOC)	3. Target specific neural plexus
4. Central Nervous System (CNS)	4. Target specific spinal segment
5. Neuromuscular/ Myofascial Trigger Point (MFTrP)	5. Target CNS (specific cerebral region/ release of specific neuropeptides)

Table III - Neuropuncture electrical techniques

Neuropuncture electrical techniques
1. Reduce inflammation and begin repair of soft tissue vs. strengthening soft tissues
2. Target specific receptors for specific neuropeptide release or specific cerebral region
3. Interrupt dysfunctional autonomic spinal reflexes
4. Change polarization of a specific nerve pathway
5. DCEA (Deep Cranial Electro Acupuncture Stimulation)/EAMS (Electrical Acupuncture Magnetic Stimulation)

Applying Western medical sciences to the classical TCM model does not subtract from the efficacy of the "traditional" acupuncture system; it only amplifies and further explains the unique, powerful neuro-modulating effects that can be scientifically understood and harnessed by Neuropuncture's techniques. From depolarizing affected nerves, targeting specific receptors for the release of specific neuropeptides, and targeting and activating specific regions of the brain for neuro-rehabilitation to regulating dysfunctional autonomic spinal reflexes, Neuropuncture will take your practice and acupuncture's future where it belongs—in the middle of mainstream medicine as opposed to on the outskirts.

As you read this book, you will notice that the Neuropuncture treatment prescriptions may include solely Neuropuncture body points or a combination of Neuropuncture body point prescriptions with Neuropuncture auricular and scalp prescriptions. This is an example of the integration of the complete Neuropuncture system, the Neuropuncture body, Neuropuncture auricular and Neuropuncture scalp systems, to better neuromodulate the patient's entire nervous system back into health. The Neuropuncture auricular system is a simple neuroanatomical system. It utilizes neuroanatomy, neurophysiology, special objective clinical assessments and direct needling techniques as does the Neuropuncture scalp system. By integrating Neuropuncture body, auricular, and scalp systems to create neural signatures that fully modulate the nervous system, we correct pathology at the root.

I have received more emails then I can count in regard to electroacupuncture's procedures and safety. Topics include placements of leads, what waveform is safe, which frequency is best, what is the difference between micro- and millicurrent, and much more. I often receive questions such as "Does it matter if the red or black clip is attached to YinTang or Du20?" In short, for the placement of leads, the answer is simply that no placement specificity is required. The placement of the leads should not matter, especially if you are using the Pantheon electrostimulator. The Pantheon is an FDA-registered electrical acupuncture stimulator that is microprocessor-frequency-calibrated, with oscilloscope confirmation of a square biphasic waveform, and with multiple safety mechanisms to ensure a very safe application of clinical electrical acupuncture. The FDA declared in the 1970s that to be FDA-registered for electrical acupuncture, the waveform for EA must be a biphasic square waveform. So, if the machine you use is positively FDA-registered for electrical acupuncture, not TENS, then by FDA rule, it should be a biphasic square waveform. That basically means positive and negative function switches, alternate current and no direct current, and the polarity switches eliminating electrolysis and tissue damage. So, in practice, I personally place the red leads close to the heart and the black leads away, but that is just for aesthetics☺. As for milli- or microcurrent, we use microcurrent in Neuropuncture only for tissue repair and neural inflammation; all other Neuropuncture Rxs and clinical strategies are done with millicurrent, but both are frequency- and point-specific. This is a very brief explanation and will need further understanding and training to best apply.

Another common topic is our Neuropuncture Treatment Prescriptions (Rxs). These treatment Rxs were constructed by the creator to provide neuroscience-evidence-based, research-supported, clinically proven neuromodulating electrical acupuncture treatment Rxs for the full range of conditions. The creator feels that it is very important to utilize twenty-first-century medical sciences in today's acupuncture profession. We should apply whatever true and accurate scientific information we can to better understand our patient's condition, symptomology, and/or medical diagnosis. That is why the creator has designed the Neuropuncture clinical process (see below). If we are given a Western medical diagnosis, great! Then we can easily look up the neuropathology of the condition and focus our understanding of the Neuropuncture Trinity on the root underlying pathological tissue or dysfunctional process. If there is no medical diagnosis, then we have a vast number of different clinical strategies and medical examinations (exams) to perform to identify the root problem. We have the orthopedic neurological evaluation (ONE), physical exam, neurological exams, functional neurology, pain upon palpation exams, lab tests such as CBC, metabolic panels, and specialty lab tests for hormones or neurotransmitters. And then we have imaging such as X-rays, MRIs, CT scans, nerve velocity conduction tests, and more. After we perform or receive results on tests, we can then apply the Neuropuncture Trinity to create a Neuropuncture Rx, Neuropuncture dosage, and Neuropuncture treatment plan accordingly.

THE NEUROPUNCTURE CLINICAL PROCESS

- ▶ Western medical Dx
- ▶ TCM (T) Dx/ TCM (P) Dx
- ▶ Physical exams: Physical exams/ ONE/ PUP/ Neurological examines/ Functional Neurology
- ▶ Imaging: MRI/ fMRI/ CT scan/ X-ray/ NVC
- ▶ Lab tests: Neurotransmitter tests/ Adrenal labs/ specialty neurohormone labs/ blood work.
- ▶ *Neuropuncture Assessment*
- ▶ Combine Neuropuncture Auricular and Scalp with the Neuropuncture body system protocols.
- ▶ Axillary modalities: Tui Na, cupping, Gua Sha, Jiao, liniments, TDP, Moxa, AIT (acupuncture injection therapy), laser, herbal and functional medicine, etc.
- ▶ Fundamental Neuroscience-based body/auricular/ scalp "functional" acupuncture prescriptions.

The last item to discuss is the acupuncture point. What is it, and what truly defines it? The creator feels that the energetic model is a complete mistranslation—confusing, controversial, and yet to be confirmed. The NIH has published several studies on the location and specificity of classical acupuncture points, indicating that locations almost always differ from practitioner to practitioner and concluding that they are more like regions or units (Choi, Jiang, and Longhurst 2012). Some of the newer terms we see in recent research are *functional acupuncture points*, or *neural acupuncture units* (Zhang, Wang, and McAlonan 2012). In Neuropuncture, we refer to our points as "functional Neuropuncture acupoint units." These regions on the body are areas that contain access to a neural network that directly communicates with the central nervous system and is distributed in the skin, muscle, and connective tissues and has an effect on the local biochemistry. These are also points, or neural regions, that have been studied in research with fMRI confirmation of their activation of specific cerebral structures. Moving forward, we will refer to these commonly as "Neuropuncture acupoints" so as not to confuse the reader. The actual Neuropuncture acupoint is made up of small nerve bundles: A-delta, C fibers, III/IV muscle fibers, tiny capillaries, and all types of different nociception ends. This is a location where we can "plug in" or communicate with the CNS. The Neuropuncture acupoints are points that directly communicate with the CNS and have neuroanatomical affiliations.

So, the functional Neuropuncture acupoints have in the name the actual nerve that will be stimulated when needled, for a deeper understanding and for better needle technique. For example, the Superficial Radial Neuropuncture Point, SRNP, stimulates the superficial radial nerve when needled. The creator has renamed, relocated, and even discovered new "functional" Neuropuncture acupoints. Below is a chart to help reference and "translate" the Neuropuncture Rxs you will find throughout the case studies. Keep in mind that some of these acupoints are not exactly classical acupuncture points but are near, or regional, to the classical point. For example, the Tibial Neuropuncture Point (TNP) is regional to Spleen 6, not exactly the classical Spleen 6 location. TNP is located two inches, or four fingers, above the medial malleolus and halfway between the Achilles tendon and the posterior border of the tibia. This region gives us clear access to the tibial nerve in that area and has been confirmed to activate specific cerebral structures. Below is a short reference chart.

Supine:
- SOrNP: SupraOrbital NP: BL2-Yu Yao
- IOrNP: InfraOrbital NP: RST2
- TrFNP: Tri-Facial NP: SJ21-SI19-GB2
- GANP: Greater Auricular NP: ISJ17
- PhNP: Philtrum NP : DU26
- SRNP: Superficial Radial NP: LI4
- MNP: Median NP: PC6
- UNP: Ulnar NP: HT7
- CTrNP: Carpal Tunnel Release NP: RPC8
- LANP: Lateral Antebrachial NP: LI11
- DRNP: Deep Radial NP: LI10.5
- SNP: Saphenous NP: SP9
- ATNP: Anterior Tibialis NP: ST36
- TNP: Tibial NP: RSP6

- DPNP: Deep Peroneal NP: LV3
- VMMP: Vastus Medialis motor point: RSP10

Prone:

- GOcNP: Greater Occipital NP: BL10
- LOcNP : Lesser Occipital NP : GB20
- SANP: Spinal Accessory NP: RGB21
- HTJJ: Hua Tuo Jia Ji points
- PNP: Paraspinal NP: Back Shu's
- PSIS NP: Posterior Sacral Illiac Spine NP (cluneal nerves): RYao Yan
- MPNP: Medial Popliteal NP: BL40
- CPNP: Common Peroneal NP: PGB34:
- SrNP: Sural NP: BL57
- PMP: Piriformis motor point
- GlutMP: Gluteus Maximus motor point

Reference table

- NP=Neuropuncture point
- R=regional
- I=inferior
- P=posterior
- MP=muscle motor points
- For case study's Rx:
- (B)=bilateral points
- (R)=right side
- (L)=left side

Throughout this book, you may come across several Neuropuncture terms that may not be clear to you. I apologize for this as it is meant not to confuse you but to introduce you to a new language in the authors' attempt to bring Neuropuncture—and acupuncture, to the forefront of medicine. If you find yourself having difficulty placing the definition of such terms in their context, then please refer to *Neuropuncture: A Clinical Handbook of Neuroscience Acupuncture, Second Edition* or the Neuropuncture website (Neuropuncture.com). For further information, Neuropuncture training, please inquire about the Neuropuncture online training platform: NeuroLab.

References

Choi, Emma, Fang Jiang, and John Longhurst. 2012. "Point specificity in acupuncture." Chinese Medicine 7, no. 4 (February 28). doi: 10.1186/1749-8546-7-4.

Zhang, Zhang-Jin, Xiao-Min Wang, and Grainne McAlonan. 2012. "Neural Acupuncture Unit: A New Concept for Interpreting Effects and Mechanisms of Acupuncture." *Evidence-Based Complementary and Alternative Medicine*, (March 8). doi: 10.1155/2012/429412.

Use of This Book

Below is the general outline and structure for each topic and case study:

1. Overview of medical condition/ medical statistics/ symptomatology.
2. Detailed neuropathophysiology description for each medical condition.
3. Neuropuncture Twenty-First-Century Medical Mindset
4. Neuropuncture Trinity for each condition (only **BOLD** sections apply)
5. Neuropuncture Treatment Rx
   a. Neuropuncture Rx (Main Neuropuncture Prescription)
   b. Neuropuncture Dosage
   c. Neuropuncture Treatment Plan
6. Case studies for each condition
7. Research, publications, references

CHAPTER ONE

Mental Health: Anxiety Disorder

Overview

Experiencing occasional anxiety is a normal part of life (Mayo clinic). There are many beneficial aspects of healthy fear and anxiety in our daily lives. Fear gives us strength to face immediate danger and motivates us to achieve; anxiety helps us to prepare for future danger and react to situations with stronger understanding (Harriman 2015). However, excessive and persistent worry and fear may involve repeated episodes of sudden feelings of intense fear that can reach a peak within minutes (panic attacks) (Martin, Ressler, Binder, and Nemeroff 2009). These feelings of anxiety and panic interfere with daily activities, are difficult to control and out of proportion to the actual danger, sometimes can last a long time. Examples of anxiety disorders include generalized anxiety disorder, social anxiety disorder (social phobia, specific phobias, and separation anxiety disorder) *(Mayo Clinic)*.

Anxiety disorders are the most common mental illness in the US, affecting 40 million adults age eighteen and older. People with this condition are three to five times more likely to go to the doctor and six times more likely to be hospitalized for psychiatric disorders than those who do not suffer from anxiety disorders. Anxiety disorders develop from a complex set of risk factors, including genetics, brain chemistry, personality, and life events (ADAA).

Signs and Symptoms

- Feeling nervous, restless, or tense
- Having a sense of impending danger, panic, or doom
- Breathing rapidly with increased heart rate
- Sweating
- Trembling
- Feeling weak or tired
- Having trouble concentrating or thinking about anything other than the present worry
- Having trouble sleeping
- Experiencing gastrointestinal (GI) problems

(Mayo Clinic)

Risk Factors

- **Trauma:** children who endured abuse or trauma or witnessed traumatic events are at higher risk of developing an anxiety disorder at some point in life. Adults who experience a traumatic event also can develop anxiety disorders.

- **Stress due to an illness:** having a health condition or serious illness can cause significant worry about issues such as your treatment and your future.
- **Stress buildup:** a bit of an event or a buildup of smaller stressful life situations may trigger excessive anxiety.
- **Personality:** people with certain personality types are more prone to anxiety disorders.
- **Other mental health disorders:** people with other mental health disorders, such as depression, often have an anxiety disorder.
- **Drugs or alcohol:** drug or alcohol use or misuse or withdrawal can cause or worsen anxiety.

(Mayo Clinic)

Complications

- Depression (which often occurs with an anxiety disorder) or other mental health disorders
- Substance abuse
- Trouble sleeping (insomnia)
- Digestive or bowel problems
- Headaches and chronic pain
- Social isolation
- Problems functioning at school or work
- Overall poor quality of life
- Suicide

(Mayo Clinic)

Neuropathophysiology of Anxiety Disorder

Anxiety is a reaction to stress that has both psychological and physical features. The feeling is thought to arise in the amygdala, a brain region that is part of the limbic system and governs many intense emotional responses. The function of the amygdala is to assess the emotional significance of things that happen in your environment. Particularly, it assesses whether or not something in your environment is a threat to you and, if it recognizes a threat, initiates the fight or flight response. The fight and flight responses are healthy for our survival and safety; however, if the fight and flight response remain switched on, it becomes prolonged anxiety (Harriman 2015). The source of fear and anxiety is the brain. It is characterized by a variety of neuroendocrine, neurotransmitter, and neuroanatomical disruptions. The prefrontal cortex (PFC) is responsible for decision making, planning, and predicting consequences for potential behaviors. The ventromedial PFC controls impulses and regulates mood. Research has found that when anxiety disorders are left untreated, the dorsomedial PFC, anterior cingulate, hippocampus, dorsolateral PFC, and orbito PFC all appear to decrease in size. The longer the anxiety goes untreated, the smaller and weaker they appear to be (Martin, Binder, and Nemeroff 2009).

The amygdala initiates the brain processes that create both fear and anxiety when facing a threat. It sends a signal to another part of the brain called the hypothalamus. It then activates the pituitary gland and then the adrenal gland. This encompasses the HPA (hypothalamus-pituitary-adrenal) axis. The adrenal gland secretes the hormones—adrenaline, noradrenaline, and cortisol. These hormones trigger a number of changes in the body: heartbeats increase, breathing is faster, face feels flushed, blood pressure increases, the amount of sugar in the blood increases, blood flows away from the digestive tract, and blood flow to the muscles increases to prepare to take action. When the anxiety becomes chronic, the brain begins to produce excess fear-related neurotransmitters, such as adrenaline, while reducing production of neurotransmitters associated with happiness and relaxation such as dopamine and serotonin. When the body is low in serotonin, there are a few common symptoms, including difficulty sleeping, muscle aches, fatigue, headaches, frequent nightmares, excessive worrying, and possible panic attacks with rapid heart rate, sweating, shaking, shortness of breath, dizziness, and nausea (Harriman 2015).

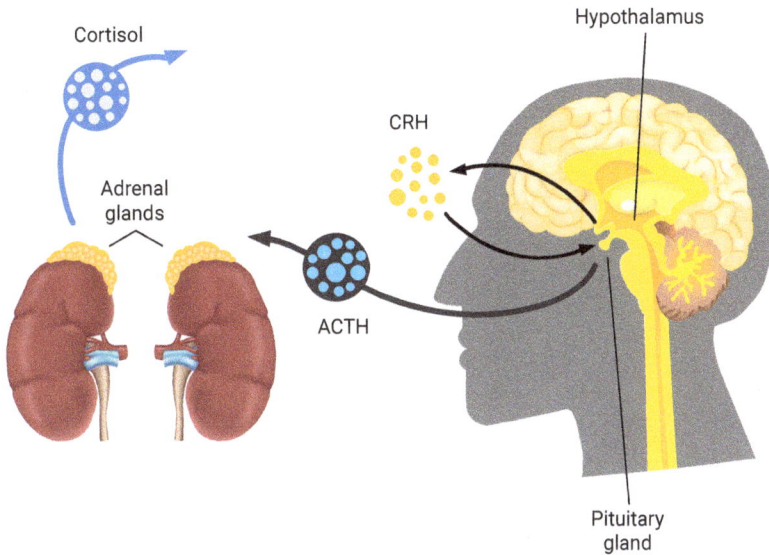

fig. 1.1.1

The brain directly responds to neurotransmitters, the chemicals that send messages to the brain. Those link to anxiety including serotonin, gamma-aminobutyric acid (GABA), norepinephrine, and dopamine. Hormones may affect anxiety as well. These hormones include adrenaline/epinephrine and thyroid hormone. Adrenaline is released when fight or flight is active, and it causes rapid heart rate, tension in the muscles, and more. However chronic anxiety may damage the ability to control adrenaline and lead to further anxiety symptoms. Thyroid hormone regulates the amount of serotonin, GABA, and norepinephrine produced and distributed to the brain. (Martin, Ressler, Binder, and Nemeroff 2009).

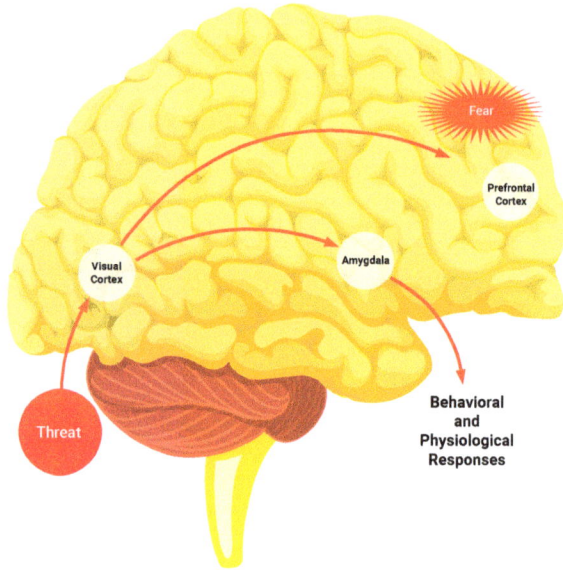

fig. 1.1.2

Neuropuncture's Twenty-First-Century Medical Mindset

Target specific regions of the brain to neuromodulate the stress hormone levels (cortisol) and neuro-rehabilitate the amygdala and ventromedial prefrontal cortex back into health; target specific receptors for specific neuropeptide release—dopamine, serotonin, GABA, and benzodiazepine neurochemistry; neuro-regulate the HPA axis; and reduce neuronal excitability throughout the autonomic nervous system. Overall, calm the fight or flight autonomic nervous system and reduce overall stress on the brain, heart, and muscles.

Table II - Neuropuncture mechanisms and treatment principles

Neuropuncture neurophysiological mechanisms	Neuropuncture treatment principles
1. Local effect	1. Harness local effect
2. Spinal segmental	2. Target specific nerve
3. Endogenous Opioid Circuit (EOC)	3. Target specific neural plexus
4. Central Nervous System (CNS)	4. Target specific spinal segment
5. Neuromuscular/ Myofascial Trigger Point (MFTrP)	**5. Target CNS (specific cerebral region/ release of specific neuropeptides)**

Table III - Neuropuncture electrical techniques

Neuropuncture electrical techniques
1. Reduce inflammation and begin repair of soft tissue vs. strengthening soft tissues
2. **Target specific receptors for specific neuropeptide release or specific cerebral region**
3. Interrupt dysfunctional autonomic spinal reflexes
4. Change polarization of a specific nerve pathway
5. DCEA (Deep Cranial Electro Acupuncture Stimulation)/EAMS (Electrical Acupuncture Magnetic Stimulation)

Table 1: Neuropuncture prescription - anxiety disorder

NEUROPUNCTURE PRESCRIPTION	
Condition	Anxiety Rx
Neuropuncture Rx	1) *NADA: Shenmen (*DE)-Tranquilizer (*OE): EA 2) Sishencong-Anmien(B) 3)TNP(B)
EA Lead Placement	Use one lead in 1) connect Shenmen in *DE to Tranquilizer point in the *OE (ear to ear). 2) Use two leads for Sishencong-Anmien on each side of the head. 3) Use one lead for TNP; connect bilaterally
Neuropuncture Dosage	1) @2 Hz millicurrent for up to 45 minutes 2)&3) @ 2–4 Hz millicurrent for 25–30 minutes. Apply 2x/week for 6 weeks.
Commentary	This prescription targets regions of the brain for neuro-rehabilitation, while neuro-modulating the brain chemistry to reduce the present anxiety state. This Neuropuncture Rx targets dopamine, serotonin, GABA, and benzodiazepine, while reducing cortisol and regulating the HPA axis.

*NADA: Shenmen, sympathetic, kidney, liver, lung

*DE= dominant ear   *OE= other ear

The following cases had the Neuropuncture anxiety Rx performed with varying treatment plans.

CASE STUDY #1
Submitted by Dr. Michael C., FL

Patient Gender: Male

Patient Age: 34

Patient Chief Complaint and Main Symptomatology: Extreme stress and anxiety with insomnia for past 1.3 years

History of Chief Complaint: Anxiety, leading to minor depression

Onset (O) 2013, divorced with two children. Experiences an extreme amount of daily stress. Patient is an entrepreneur, manages several private businesses.

S/s: Patient always feels like a rush of adrenaline; he experiences an "edgy" feeling constantly

Suffers from lack of energy, shortness of breath (SOB), hands get sweaty, his vision is affected, bright lights are irritating.

Patient complains of low-back pain, stiff and sore neck, as well as sore and painful feet.

Bowel Movement (BM): not diarrhea, but loose with stress; undigested food

Western medical diagnosis (Dx): IBS.

Prescription Medications: None

Supplements and Herbs: Multivitamins, 28-day metabolic detoxification program from Metagenics.

TCM Diagnosis—Tongue and Pulse:

- Tongue: thick white coat

- Pulse: weak and soft

Significant Previous Relevant Treatment History: Patient has never tried acupuncture before.

Intervention: The Neuropuncture Anxiety Rx was performed in a 12 Neuropuncture treatment plan of 2 sessions per week for 6 weeks.

Results from Neuropuncture Treatment:

Patient reported a marked reduction in anxiety and improved sleep after a single treatment, with 100 percent reduction in anxiety after nine sessions. He actually had to be reminded that his first chief complaint was anxiety at the final session. Patient was able to complete his daily multiple business tasks without overwhelming stress and he reported sleeping seven to nine hours per night while awakening well rested.

CASE STUDY #2
Submitted by Nancy C., FL

Patient Gender: Female

Patient Age: 58

Patient Chief Complaint and Main Symptomatology: Extreme stress and anxiety

History of Chief Complaint: Patient complained of feeling "emotionally stuck" with bouts of "anxiety/depression" for six months. She has been experiencing extreme stress and anxiety for the past month as her husband was admitted in hospital several times due to medical issues. Patient has no children and lack of local family support. She has been internalizing the stress that causes feelings of "choking" and "helplessness." She also reported suffering from insomnia at night.

Prescription Medications: None

Supplements and Herbs: Multivitamins

TCM Review of Systems (10 Traditional Questions):

- Fragile-looking
- Pale face
- Looks exhausted
- Eye bags

TCM Diagnosis—Tongue and Pulse:

- Tongue: thin and pale
- Pulse: deep and weak

Significant Previous Relevant Treatment History: Patient has never tried acupuncture before.

Intervention: The Neuropuncture Anxiety Rx was performed.

Results from Neuropuncture Treatment:

Patient reported after the first treatment, she felt "being lifted up" with a noticeable reduction in her stress and anxiety. She also felt more capacity to manage the stress, and, best of all, her sleep was improved, and she awakes well rested.

CASE STUDY #3

Submitted by Dr. Michael C., FL

Patient Gender: Male

Patient Age: 28

Patient Chief Complaint and Main Symptomatology: Extreme anxiety associated with addiction.

History of Chief Complaint: Severe anxiety and cravings from heroin with methamphetamine addiction. Patient just confided that he did use the drug on the morning of the treatment and was currently having severe anxiety.

Prescription Medications: None

Supplements and Herbs: None

TCM Diagnosis—Tongue and Pulse:

- Tongue: thick white coat, red tip
- Pulse: tight and wiry

Significant Previous Relevant Treatment History: Patient has been in and out of drug treatment centers for past eight years.

Intervention: The Neuropuncture Anxiety Rx was performed

Results from Neuropuncture Treatment:

Patient initially laid down on the table and was visibly uncomfortable and restless. We inserted the needles and began to increase the intensity on the EA device. The practitioner was able to reach a high level of stimulation intensity, voltage, and we then told the patient to relax, that the practitioner would check on him in five to ten minutes. When practitioner returned, the patient reported a major reduction in anxiety and was smiling with eyes closed and moving his head in an affirmative motion, signaling that he was feeling much improved, with two thumbs up.

References

Anxiety and Depression Association of America. "Facts and Statistics." Retrieved April 20, 2020. https://adaa.org/about-adaa/press-room/facts-statistics.

Harriman, Garrett Ray. 2015. "Therapies for Anxiety." Explorable, June 26. https://explorable.com/e/therapies-for-anxiety?gid=21000.

Harvard Health Publishing: Harvard Medical School. "Pain, anxiety, and depression." Updated June 5, 2019. https://www.health.harvard.edu/staying-healthy/anxiety_and_physical_illness.

Maron, E. and D. Nutt. 2017. "Biological markers of generalized anxiety disorder." *Dialogues in Clinical Neuroscience* 19, no. 2 (June):147–157.

Martin, E., K. Ressler, E. Binder, and C. Nemeroff. 2009. "The Neurobiology of Anxiety Disorders: Brain Imaging, Genetics, and Psychoneuroendocrinology," *Psychiatric Clinics of North America* 32, no. 3, (September):549–575. Doi:10:1016/j.psc.2009.05.004.

Mayo Clinic. "Anxiety disorders." Updated May 4, 2018. https://www.mayoclinic.org/diseases-conditions/anxiety/symptoms-causes/syc-20350961.

National Institute of Mental Health, "Any Anxiety Disorder." Updated November 2017. https://www.nimh.nih.gov/health/statistics/any-anxiety-disorder.shtml.

Mental Health: Depression

Overview

Depression is a common but serious mood disorder that impacts the lives of millions of children and adults around the world. It causes severe symptoms that affect how you feel, think, and handle daily activities (NIH). Depression is a crippling mental illness that undermines a person's sense of motivation, purpose, and self-worth. It is not known exactly what causes depression. As with many mental disorders, a variety of factors may be involved, such as biological differences. People with depression appear to have physical changes to their brain, or it can result from imbalanced brain chemistry of specific neurotransmitters alterations. It could be hormone imbalance that triggers depression, or it could be due to inherited traits (Mayo Clinic).

According to the National Institute of Health, approximately 17.3 million adults in the US have had at least one major depressive episode in their lives. The prevalence of major depressive episodes is higher among adult females compared to males and is highest among individuals age eighteen to twenty-five.

Signs and Symptoms

If you have been experiencing some of the following signs and symptoms most of the day, nearly every day, for at least two weeks, you may be suffering from depression:

- Persistent sadness, anxiety, tearfulness, or emptiness
- Feelings of hopelessness or pessimism
- Irritability, angry outbursts, and frustration, even over small matters
- Feelings of guilt, worthlessness, or helplessness
- Loss of interest or pleasure in most or all normal activities
- Tiredness and lack of energy, so even small tasks take extra effort
- Feeling restless or having trouble sitting still
- Difficulty concentrating, remembering, or making decisions
- Difficulty sleeping, early morning awakening, or oversleeping
- Appetite and/or weight changes
- Thoughts of death or suicide or suicide attempts
- Unexplained aches or pains, headaches, cramps, or digestive problems without a clear physical cause and/or that do not ease even with treatment

Not everyone who is depressed experiences every symptom. Some people experience only a few symptoms, while others may experience many.

(NIH, Mayo Clinic)

Risk Factors

- Certain personality traits, such as low self-esteem and being too dependent, self-critical, or pessimistic
- Traumatic or stressful events, such as physical or sexual abuse, the death or loss of a loved one, a difficult relationship, or financial problems
- Genetics: blood relatives with a history of depression, bipolar disorder, alcoholism, or suicide
- History of other mental health disorders, such as anxiety disorders, eating disorders, or post-traumatic stress disorder
- Abuse of alcohol or recreational drugs
- Serious or chronic illness, including cancer, stroke, chronic pain, or heart disease
- Certain medications, such as some high-blood-pressure medications or sleeping pills

(Mayo Clinic)

Complications

- Excess weight or obesity, which can lead to heart disease and diabetes
- Pain or physical illness
- Alcohol or drug abuse
- Anxiety, panic disorder, or social phobia
- Family conflicts, relationship difficulties, and work or school problems

- Social isolation
- Suicidal feelings, suicide attempts, or suicide
- Premature death from medical conditions

(Mayo Clinic)

Neuropathophysiology of Depression

The prefrontal cortex (PFC), dorsolateral prefrontal cortex (DLPFC), amygdala, and particularly the hippocampus are the brain structures most widely studied in relation to depression. Magnetic resonance studies show a reduction in the brain volume of depressed patients, with large volume reductions in the anterior cingulate cortex and orbitofrontal cortex and moderate reduction in the hippocampus. The amygdala is involved in emotional learning and memory. The hippocampus is the most widely studied brain structure in relation to depression. It is rich in corticosteroid receptors and is closely linked to the hypothalamus, providing regulatory feedback to the HPA axis (Palazidou 2012).

There are three major regions of the brain that show abnormality in depression from published literature of brain imaging studies: 1) cortical abnormalities include prefrontal cortex, cingulate cortex, orbital frontal cortex, and the insula; 2) subcortical limbic brain regions include amygdala, hippocampus, and the dorsomedial thalamus; 3) basal ganglia and brainstem. In summary, various cortical, subcortical, and brainstem regions have been shown to have abnormal activation or metabolism in brain imaging studies (Pandya, M. et al. 2012).

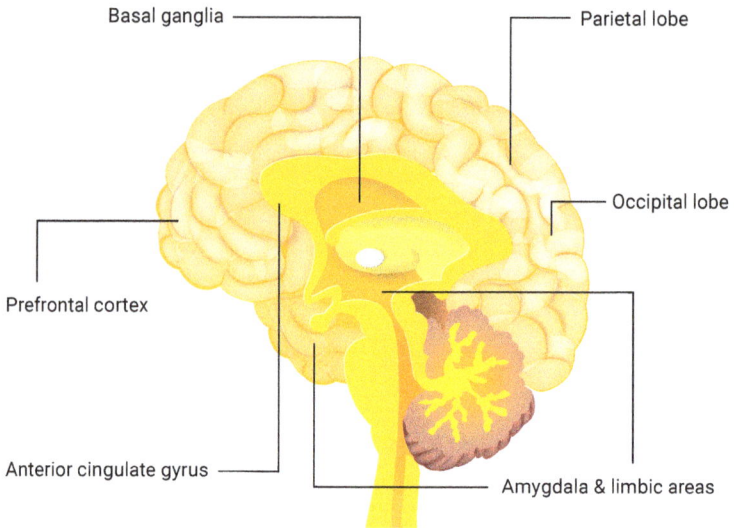

Basal ganglia — Parietal lobe
Occipital lobe
Prefrontal cortex
Anterior cingulate gyrus — Amygdala & limbic areas

fig. 1.2.3

*Notice the lack of cortical engagement and lack of activity in specific cerebral regions in the patients with depression. This illustrates that it is not a single region of the brain but a neural signature that connects and engages multiple cerebral regions.

New image of MRI and brain:

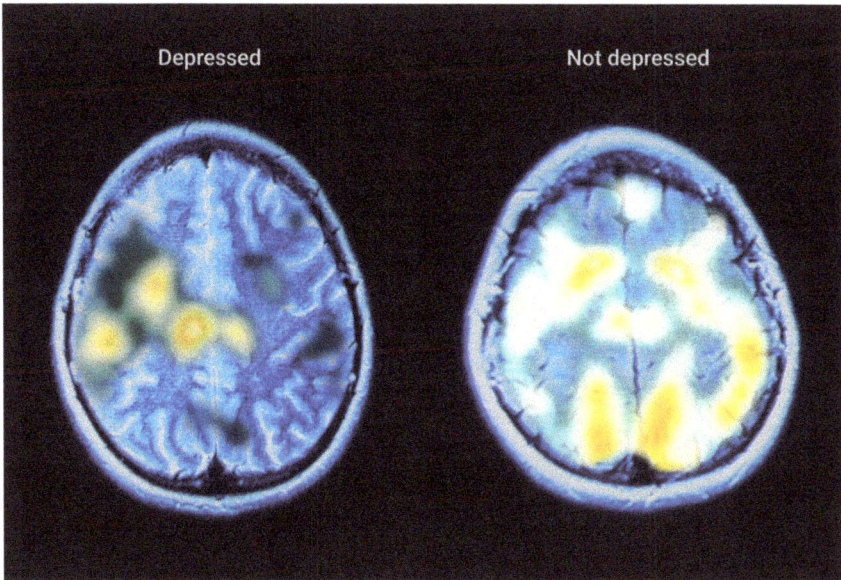

fig. 1.2.4

Immunological mechanisms have also been implicated in the complex pathophysiology of depression. It has been suggested that impaired glucocorticoid receptor function may be related to chronic exposure to inflammatory cytokines associated with chronic physical illness. Both the noradrenergic and serotonergic pathways project from their midbrain nuclei into the limbic and prefrontal area and the hippocampus. The hippocampus is rich in brain-derived neurotrophic factor (BDNF), which plays a major role in neuronal growth, survival, and maturation as well as synaptic plasticity in the adult brain. Stress suppresses BDNF synthesis in the hippocampus (Palazidou 2012).

Neuropuncture's Twenty-First-Century Medical Mindset

Neuromodulate dopamine and serotonin levels in the brain. Target specific regions of the brain to neuro-rehabilitate them: the prefrontal dorsolateral cortex, amygdala, hippocampus; target specific receptors—D1 and 5HTP receptors—for specific neuropeptide release of dopamine and serotonin, also increasing the production of BDNF and GDNF (glial derivative neurotropic factor); regulate hormones via HPA axis. Increase the cellular energy and ATP production to increase overall energy.

Table II - Neuropuncture mechanisms and treatment principles

Neuropuncture neurophysiological mechanisms	Neuropuncture treatment principles
1. Local effect	1. Harness local effect
2. Spinal segmental	2. Target specific nerve
3. Endogenous Opioid Circuit (EOC)	3. Target specific neural plexus
4. Central Nervous System (CNS)	4. Target specific spinal segment
5. Neuromuscular/ Myofascial Trigger Point (MFTrP)	**5. Target CNS (specific cerebral region/ release of specific neuropeptides)**

Table III - Neuropuncture electrical techniques

Neuropuncture electrical techniques

1. Reduce inflammation and begin repair of soft tissue vs. strengthening soft tissues

2. **Target specific receptors for specific neuropeptide release or specific cerebral region**

3. Interrupt dysfunctional autonomic spinal reflexes

4. Change polarization of a specific nerve pathway

5. **DCEA (Deep Cranial Electro Acupuncture Stimulation)/EAMS (Electrical Acupuncture Magnetic Stimulation)**

Table 2: Neuropuncture prescription - depression

NEUROPUNCTURE PRESCRIPTION	
Condition	Clinical Depression Rx
Neuropuncture Rx	1) Du20–Yintang: EA 2) TNP(B): EA 3) St8-Sishencong (B): EA
EA Lead Placement	1) Attach one lead from Yintang to Du20. 2) use one lead to connect TNP bilaterally 3) use two leads, one on each side connect St8 to Sishencong
Neuropuncture Dosage	EA: 2-4 Hz millicurrent for 25 minutes, 2 times a week for 6 weeks=12 sessions or 3 times a week for 4 weeks=12 sessions.
Commentary	This is a combination of prescriptions to have a collective, cumulative effect on the nervous system. Part of this protocol has been published in many separate medical publications, and they always state how it is effective on the metabolism of medication, specifically SSRIs. It targets the PFC and DLPFC of the D1 dopamine receptors as well as the 5HTP receptor of the hypothalamus for serotonin and increases the production of BDNF and GDNF. Also, hippocampal activation for negative memories. In addition, the TNP aspect is for cellular energy support, since most patients with depression seem to lack energy. Also, TNPs support neuroendocrine regulation.

Note: The following cases had the Neuropuncture Depression Rx performed with varying treatment plans.

CASE STUDY #1
Submitted by Dr. Michael C., FL

Patient Gender: Female
Patient Age: 38

Patient Chief Complaint and Main Symptomatology: Severe depression, dizziness, and sleep issues

History of Chief Complaint: Onset of depression was during childhood, entire life with emotional "ups and downs." No suicidal ideologies or plans; more constant "blues." Bad head injury as a child but no diagnosis. Recently, blues became really "bad"—patient presented tearful and depressed. Patient also reported a lack of motivation. Dizziness began 1.5 months ago. Patient tried a juice fast for two weeks, but she became dizzier and anxious, so stopped the juice fast. Her uncle is a homeopathic doctor, and he prescribed drops, but they also created more depression.

Prescription Medications: None (but next step was to begin taking prescription medications)

Supplements and Herbs: Multivitamins

TCM Review of Systems (10 Traditional Questions):

- Energy: 5/10—if no sleep 1–2/10
- Sleep: sometimes difficulty falling asleep and staying asleep: 5–7 hours per night.
- GI: not hungry, nervous—thirsty, dry mouth
- BM: 2+, usually constipated; 1x day.
- Emotions: No motivation or happiness.
- Digestion was fine; hungry, usually hunger, no appetite.

TCM Diagnosis—Tongue and Pulse:

- Tongue: thin coat and pale, swollen body
- Pulse: deep and weak

Significant Previous Relevant Treatment History: Patient has tried prescriptions medications and counseling in the past. Nothing at this time.

Intervention: The Neuropuncture Depression Rx was performed in a 12 Neuropuncture treatment plan of 2 sessions per week for 6 weeks:

Results from Neuropuncture Treatment:

As the treatments progressed, patient reported feeling increasingly more motivated and less "blues." Patient reported 95 percent reduction in her depression in twelve sessions and no longer contemplating taking prescription medication. Dizziness cleared up after third session, and sleep improved to a regular seven hours per night. Follow-up in six months reported patient was feeling "great" and motivated.

CASE STUDY #2
Submitted by Dr. Alvaro T., FL

Patient Gender: Male
Patient Age: 37

Patient Chief Complaint and Main Symptomatology: Severe depression, diagnosed as medication-resistant depression, with history of ECT (electroconvulsive therapy). Patient had in the last twelve-month a major flare-up of his depression. He was unable to work full time (patient was only able to work two hours a day), family life was very stressful for him, and he could not stay a long time with his children which resulted in emotional and psychological fatigue and stress.

History of Chief Complaint: Struggled all his life with depression. Gained excessive weight recently. Easily stressed, and emotionally impatient. Side effect from the ECT, patient experienced reduced memory and focus.

Prescription Medications: Deplin 15 mg, Vyvanse 70 mg, Effexor 225 mg, Adderall 20 mg, Abilify 15 mg

Supplements and Herbs: None

TCM Review of Systems (10 Traditional Questions):

- Weight gain

- Heartburn

- However, sleeping through the night

TCM Diagnosis—Tongue and Pulse:

- Tongue: white body, thin coat; sublingual vein.

- Pulse: 83 bpm, slippery (L), (R) deep.

Significant Previous Relevant Treatment History: Patient has tried multiple prescription medications and counseling. Patient also has had several rounds of ECT (electroconvulsive therapy).

Intervention: The Neuropuncture Depression Rx was performed three times a week for the first two weeks then twice a week for several weeks thereafter.

Results from Neuropuncture Treatment:

Throughout the Neuropuncture treatment plan, patient was gradually improving. After the last treatment, patient was approximately 70 percent improved. Treatment stopped and follow up in 8 weeks patient reported he was now working full time, very motivated, enjoying his time with his family, and completing his DLAs (daily living activities). A 180-degree turnaround, with no depression! This is a great example of the brain demonstrating neuroplastic changes and healing continuing after the Neuropuncture treatments.

References

Mayo Clinic. 2018. "Depression (major depressive disorder)." Updated February 3, 2018. https://www.mayoclinic.org/diseases-conditions/depression/symptoms-causes/syc-20356007.

National Institute of General Medical Sciences. "Circadian Rhythms." Retrieved April 2, 2020. https://nigms.nih.gov/education/fact-sheets/Pages/Circadian-Rhythms.aspx.

National Institute of Mental Health. 2018. "Depression." February 2018. https://www.nimh.nih.gov/health/topics/depression/index.shtml.

National Institute of Mental Health. 2019. "Major Depression." February 2019. https://www.nimh.nih.gov/health/statistics/major-depression.shtml.

Palazidou, E. 2012. "The neurobiology of depression." *British Medical Bulletin* 101:127–145. Doi:10.1093/bmb/lds004.

Pandya, M., Altinay, M., Malone, D., & Anand, A. (2012). "Where in the brain is depression?" *Curr Psychiatry Rep*. December; 14(6):634–642.

World Health Organization. 2020. "Depression." Updated January 30, 2020. https://www.who.int/news-room/fact-sheets/detail/depression.

CHAPTER TWO

Orthopedic and Pain Management: Carpal Tunnel Syndrome

Overview

Carpal tunnel syndrome (CTS) is one of the most common problems affecting the hand. People with this condition may feel pain, numbness, and general weakness in the hand and wrist (Cleveland Clinic). The symptoms can be extreme and develop into lack of function or loss of use with the affected hand(s). It happens when there is increased pressure within the wrist on a nerve called the median nerve. This nerve provides sensation to the thumb, index, and middle fingers and to half of the ring finger. The small finger (the "pinky") is typically not affected (NIH). It is estimated more than 8 million people are affected by carpal tunnel syndrome each year. Surgery for CTS is the second most common type of musculoskeletal surgery (back surgery is number one), with well over 230,000 procedures performed annually. Sometimes it requires multiple surgeries, which can cause complications ranging from scar tissue overgrowth to surgical injuries (Carpal Tunnel Surgery).

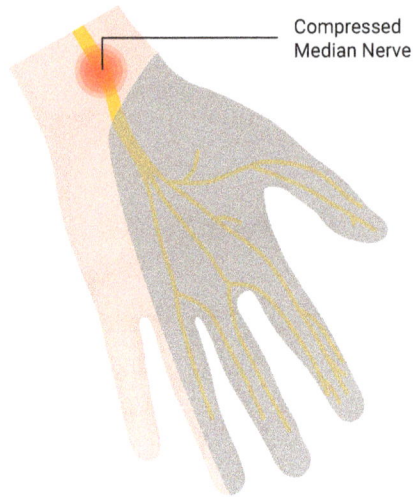

Compressed
Median Nerve

fig. 2.1.1

Signs and Symptoms

- Numbness at night
- Tingling and/or pain in the fingers (especially the thumb, index, and middle fingers
- Waking up at night from sleep
- Decreased feeling in the fingertips
- Difficulty using the hand for small tasks
- Weakness in the hand
- Inability to perform tasks that require delicate motions (such as buttoning a shirt)
- Dropping objects
- In the most severe conditions, the muscles at the base of the thumb visibly shrink in size (atrophy)

(NIH)

Risk Factors

- **Anatomic factors:** a wrist fracture or dislocation or arthritis
- **Gender:** women are three times more likely than men to develop CTS
- **Nerve-damaging conditions:** diabetes increases risk of nerve damage
- **Inflammation conditions:** rheumatoid arthritis and other inflammatory conditions can affect the lining around the tendons and put pressure on the median nerve
- **Medications:** use of Arimidex may link to CTS
- **Obesity:** increases risk
- **Body fluid changes:** fluid retention may increase risk
- **Other medical conditions:** menopause, thyroid disorders, kidney failure, and lymphedema may increase risk
- **Workplace factors:** vibrating tools, assembly lines, and computer mouse use may increase risk

(Mayo Clinic)

Complications

- Carpal tunnel syndrome may continue to increase median nerve damage, leading to permanent impairment and disability
- Some individuals can develop chronic wrist and hand pain (with or without sympathetic dystrophy).

Neuropathophysiology of Carpal Tunnel Syndrome

The carpal tunnel is a narrow canal or tube in the wrist. This part of the wrist allows the median nerve and tendons to connect the hand and forearm. The tunnel includes carpal bones and a ligament. The carpal bones make up the bottom and sides of the tunnel. They are formed in a semicircle. The top of the tunnel is the ligament that holds the tunnel together. Inside the tunnel are the median nerve and tendons. The median nerve provides sensation to most of the fingers in the hand except the little finger. It also adds strength to the base of the thumbs and index finger. Carpal tunnel syndrome is caused when the carpal tunnel in the wrist narrows. This presses down on the median nerve and tendons and makes them swell, which cuts off sensation in the fingers and hand (NIH).

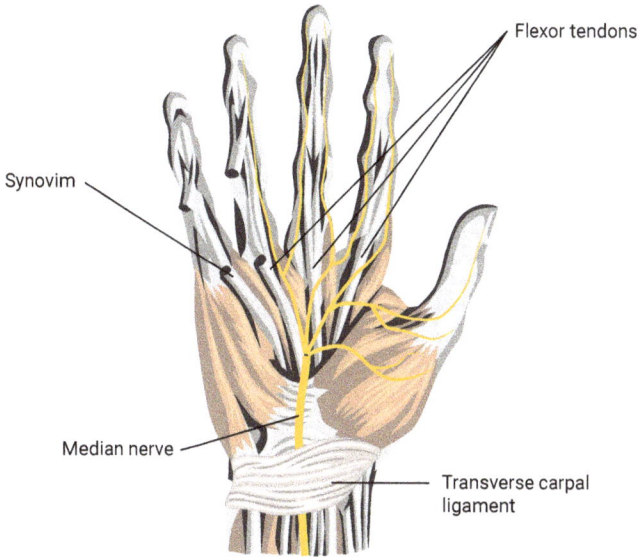

Flexor tendons

Synovim

Median nerve

Transverse carpal ligament

fig. 2.1.2

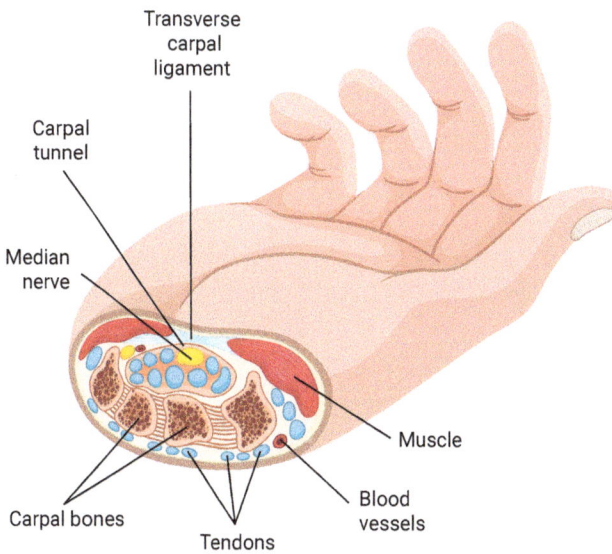

Transverse carpal ligament

Carpal tunnel

Median nerve

Muscle

Carpal bones

Tendons

Blood vessels

fig. 2.1.3

Neuropuncture's Twenty-First-Century Medical Mindset

Target the median nerve and the carpal tunnel to reduce inflammation and repair the neuromuscular damage, while stimulating the endogenous opioid circuit for pain management. Then neuro-regulate and neuro-rehabilitate the median nerve, carpal tunnel, and carpal tunnel ligament back to health.

Table II - Neuropuncture mechanisms and treatment principles

Neuropuncture neurophysiological mechanisms	Neuropuncture treatment principles
1. Local effect	**1. Harness local effect**
2. Spinal segmental	**2. Target specific nerve**
3. Endogenous Opioid Circuit (EOC)	3. Target specific neural plexus
4. Central Nervous System (CNS)	4. Target specific spinal segment
5. Neuromuscular/ Myofascial Trigger Point (MFTrP)	**5. Target CNS (specific cerebral region/ release of specific neuropeptides)**

Table III - Neuropuncture electrical techniques

Neuropuncture electrical techniques

1. **Reduce inflammation and begin repair of soft tissue vs. strengthening soft tissues**

2. **Target specific receptors for specific neuropeptide release or specific cerebral region**

3. Interrupt dysfunctional autonomic spinal reflexes

4. **Change polarization of a specific nerve pathway**

5. DCEA (Deep Cranial Electro Acupuncture Stimulation)/EAMS (Electrical Acupuncture Magnetic Stimulation)

Table 3: Neuropuncture prescription - carpal tunnel syndrome

NEUROPUNCTURE PRESCRIPTION	
Condition	Carpal Tunnel Syndrome Rx
Neuropuncture Rx	1) CTrNP-MNP: EA (only on the affected side; motor points of forearm muscles can also be added.)
EA Lead Placement	Use one lead to attach the black clip on the CTrNP (carpal tunnel release NP) and attach the red clip to the MNP on the affected side.
Neuropuncture Dosage	EA: Begin with 25 Hz microcurrent for 25–30 minutes; Then gradually increase millicurrent to 2 Hz if needed. Apply 2x a week for 3 weeks
Commentary	This prescription directly targets the median nerves and the carpal tunnel and aids in the reduction of inflammation and soft tissue repair locally.

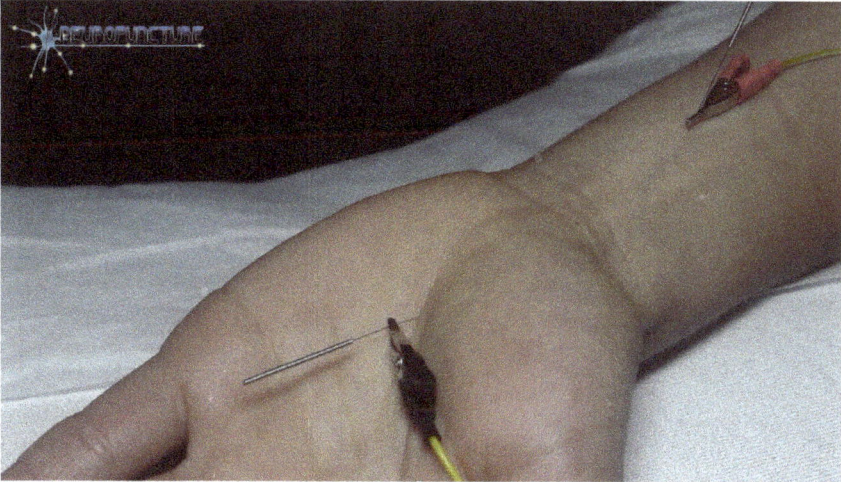

fig. 2.1.4

Note: The following cases had the Neuropuncture Carpal Tunnel Syndrome Rx performed with varying treatment plans.

CASE STUDY #1
Submitted by Dr. Michael C., FL

Patient Gender: Male
Patient Age: 59

Patient Chief Complaint and Main Symptomatology: Severe bilateral carpal tunnel syndrome.

History of Chief Complaint:

Patient presents with severe bilateral hand, wrist, and forearm pain, swelling, and stiffness. Patient sustained a work-related injury damaging his carpal tunnel that resulted in multiple bilateral wrist surgeries. Patient presents with +4 PUP (pain upon palpation), reduced ROM of flexion and extension of the wrist with severe visible swelling and stiffness.

Prescription Medications: Norco, gabapentin 300 mg 2x, Vicodin 7.5

Supplements and Herbs: Multivitamins

TCM Diagnosis—Tongue and Pulse:

- Tongue: swollen and pale
- Pulse: deep and weak

Significant Previous Relevant Treatment History: Patient has had surgery, cortisone injections, and prescription pain medications.

Intervention: The Neuropuncture CTS Rx was performed in a 8 Neuropuncture treatment plan of 2 sessions per week for 4 weeks:

Results from Neuropuncture Treatment: Patient finished his eight-session treatment plan with 75 percent reduction in pain and was able to remove one narcotic prescription (Vicodin) and reduce his gabapentin by half. He was able to open doors and shake hands again. The treatments have lessened his pain significantly, reduced the swelling, increased his daily activities, increased his ROM, and improved his quality of life. His hands, forearms, and wrists show significant benefits with the Neuropuncture treatment.

References

Cleveland Clinic. "Carpal Tunnel Syndrome." Cleveland Clinic. Retrieved April 3, 2020. https://my.clevelandclinic.org/health/diseases/4005-carpal-tunnel-syndrome.

National Institute of Neurological Disorders and Strokes, "Carpal Tunnel Syndrome Fact Sheet." Retrieved April 3, 2020. https://www.ninds.nih.gov/Disorders/Patient-Caregiver-Education/Fact-Sheets/Carpal-Tunnel-Syndrome-Fact-Sheet.

The Carpal Solution. "Risks and Complications of Carpal Tunnel Surgery." Retrieved April 3, 2020. https://www.mycarpaltunnel.com/carpal-tunnel-surgery/complications-risks/.

CHAPTER TWO
Orthopedic and Pain Management: Migraine Headache

Overview

A migraine headache can cause severe throbbing pain or a pulsing sensation, usually on one side of the head. It is often accompanied by nausea, vomiting, and extreme sensitivity to light and sound. Migraine headache attacks can last for hours to days, and the pain can be so severe that it interferes with your daily activities. For some people, a warning symptom known as an aura occurs before or with the headache. An aura can include visual disturbances, such as flashes of light or blind spots, or other neurological disturbances, such as tingling on one side of the face or in an arm or leg and difficulty speaking (Mayo Clinic).

Migraine is the third most common disease in the world, affecting an estimated one out of every six Americans and one in five women.

Overall, 15.3 percent of the population—9.7 percent of males and 20.7 percent of females—is affected. The prevalence has been remarkably stable over a period of nineteen years (Burch, R., 2018).

Signs and Symptoms: Migraine often begins in childhood, adolescence, or early adulthood and can progress through four stages: prodrome, aura, attack, and postdrome. Not everyone who has migraine goes through all stages.

Prodrome: one or two days before a migraine, you might notice

- Constipation
- Mood changes, from depression to euphoria
- Food cravings
- Neck stiffness
- Increased thirst and urination
- Frequent yawning

Aura

- Visual phenomena, such as seeing various shapes, bright spots, or flashes of light
- Vision loss
- Pins-and-needles sensations in an arm or leg
- Weakness or numbness in the face or one side of the body
- Difficulty speaking
- Hearing noises or music
- Uncontrollable jerking or other movements

Attack

- Pain usually on one side of the head, but often on both sides
- Pain that throbs or pulses
- Sensitivity to light, sound, and sometimes smell and touch
- Nausea and vomiting

Postdrome

- Feeling drained for up to a day
- Feeling confused
- Sometimes sudden head movement might bring on the pain again.

(Mayo Clinic)

Risk Factors

- Genetic
- Stress and other emotions
- Biological and environmental conditions, such as hormonal shifts or exposure to light or smells
- Fatigue and changes in one's sleep pattern
- Weather changes
- Glaring or flickering lights
- Sleep disturbance, sleep apnea
- Certain foods and drinks

(Hopkins Medicine)

Neuropathophysiology of Migraine

Migraine is an inherited, neurological, episodic disorder involving sensory sensitivity in the brain with extremely incapacitating neurological symptoms. Studies found migraine is a complex primary brain disorder that involves a cascade of events leading to recurrent inappropriate activations of the trigeminocervical pain system. The neurophysiological events that result in the visual or sensory symptoms also result in activation of trigeminal/cervical nociceptive neurons. The convergence of cervical and trigeminal afferents explains why neck stiffness or pain is present in migraine sufferers (American Headache Society; Noseda and Burstein 2013).

Pathology of the posterior auricular nerve (also called the greater auricular nerve) will cause a parietal headache associated with ear pain. The entrapment may be seen many years after a traumatic injury and as a cicatrix of scar tissue forms around the nerve (Techniques in Regional Anesthesia and Pain Management (2005) 9, 68–72)

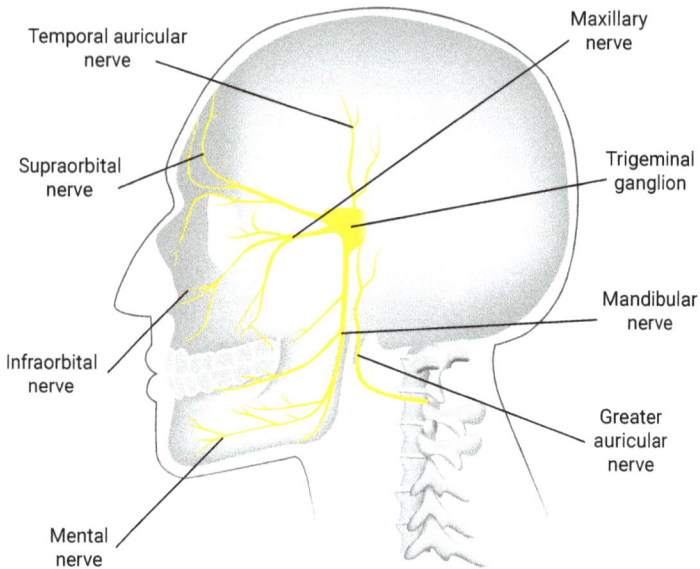

fig. 2.2.1

Seven main types of migraines

1. **Migraine without aura:** throbbing pain that starts on one side of the head (for many sufferers, migraines tend to start behind the left eye). Moving around tends to make the pain worse, and it's normal to feel nauseous, dizzy, and sensitive to light and sound.

2. **Migraine with aura:** visual disturbances before a migraine begins, followed by common migraine symptoms

3. **Menstrual migraine:** coincides with menstrual period

4. **Vestibular migraine:** vertigo, dizziness, and trouble with balance

5. **Migraine without headache:** no actual headache pain

6. **Abdominal migraine:** stomach pain instead of a headache
7. **Status migrainosus:** a migraine that lasts more than seventy-two hours

Studies have found that chemical compounds and hormones such as serotonin and estrogen often play a role in pain sensitivity for migraine sufferers. One aspect of migraine pain happens due to waves of activity by groups of excitable brain cells. These trigger chemicals, such as serotonin, that narrow blood vessels. Serotonin is a neurochemical necessary for communication between nerve cells. It can cause narrowing of blood vessels throughout the body (vasoconstriction). When serotonin or estrogen levels change, the result for some is a migraine. Serotonin levels may affect both sexes, while fluctuating estrogen levels affect women only (Goadsby 2012).

The serotonin is involved in regulating the hypothalamic-pituitary-adrenal (HPA) axis. The HPA axis is a neuroendocrine system that regulates the body's response to stress and has complex interactions with brain serotonergic, noradrenergic, and dopaminergic systems (Goadsby 2012).

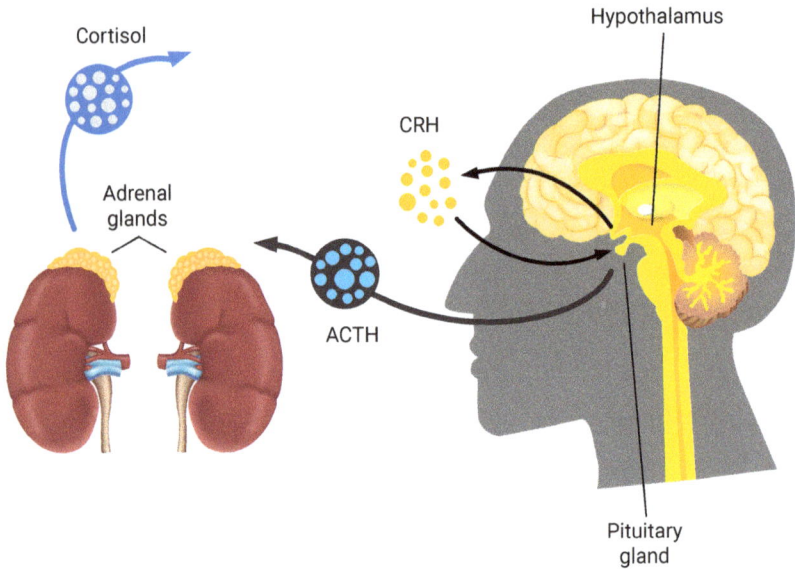

fig. 2.2.2

Neuropuncture Twenty-First-Century Medical Mindset

Target trigeminal, auriculotemporal, and the facial nerve, as well as the greater auricular nerve while neuromodulating the endogenous opioid circuit for pain management. Change the polarization of specific nerve pathways. Utilize the Neuropuncture electrical sciences to reduce neural inflammation along pathological nerves. Neuromodulate specific regions of the brain and neuro-rehabilitate them back to health while regulating the neuroendocrine system for hormone homeostasis.

Table II - Neuropuncture mechanisms and treatment principles

Neuropuncture neurophysiological mechanisms	Neuropuncture treatment principles
1. Local effect	1. Harness local effect
2. Spinal segmental	**2. Target specific nerve**
3. Endogenous Opioid Circuit (EOC)	**3. Target specific neural plexus**
4. Central Nervous System (CNS)	4. Target specific spinal segment
5. Neuromuscular/ Myofascial Trigger Point (MFTrP)	**5. Target CNS (specific cerebral region/ release of specific neuropeptides)**

Table III - Neuropuncture electrical techniques

Neuropuncture electrical techniques
1. Reduce inflammation and begin repair of soft tissue vs. strengthening soft tissues
2. Target specific receptors for specific neuropeptide release or specific cerebral region
3. Interrupt dysfunctional autonomic spinal reflexes
4. Change polarization of a specific nerve pathway
5. DCEA (Deep Cranial Electro Acupuncture Stimulation)/EAMS (Electrical Acupuncture Magnetic Stimulation)

Table 4: Neuropuncture prescription - migraines

NEUROPUNCTURE PRESCRIPTION	
Condition	Migraine Rx
Neuropuncture Rx	1) GANP-TriFNP (B): EA 2) SRNP(B):EA 3) TNP-DPNP(B): EA
EA Lead Placement	1) Use one lead to attach one clip on TriFNP and GANP, using longer needles from one side to the other side. 2) Use one lead to attach to SRNP(B). 3) Then use two leads to attach TNP-DPNP(B). Use four leads altogether
Neuropuncture Dosage	1) EA@ 25 Hz microcurrent, 2) & 3) EA@2 Hz millicurrent for 25–30 minutes. Apply 2x/week for 6 weeks.
Commentary	This Neuropuncture Rx targets the main facial nerves (trigeminal, facial, auriculotemporal nerves) and cranial nerves involved in migraine pathology as well as a neuroendocrine support for hormonal neuro-regulation.

Note: The following cases had the Neuropuncture Migraine Rx performed with varying treatment plans.

CASE STUDY #1
Submitted by Peter L., New Zealand

Patient Gender: Female
Patient Age: 16

Patient Chief Complaint and Main Symptomatology: Chronic fatigue, severe migraines, and anxiety

History of Chief Complaint:

The history of this patient's complaints started about two years prior to presenting in my clinic. The first symptoms started with insomnia and anxiety after her parents went through a difficult divorce. Shortly after this, the patient got conjunctivitis, a cold, and a chest infection that was treated with three rounds of antibiotics. This is when the migraines and vomiting started leading to the chronic fatigue.

Prescription Medications: Almotriptan, Naratriptan

Supplements and Herbs: None

TCM Review of Systems (10 Traditional Questions): Patient presents with a pale/green complexion with dark rings under her eyes. She is very thin, bruises easily, is cold to touch, and struggles to hold her head up. Her migraine frequency is four times a week on average, with constant headaches that can last for days on end and tend to be frontal, temporal, and behind the eyes with a sharp pain quality, generalized feeling of heaviness, and constant nausea. She vomits six to twelve times in every twenty-four hours, mostly during the night. This is accompanied by a tight and burning sensation in her chest and stomach. Her anxiety presents with overthinking, worry, apprehension, and avoidance. She has palpitations, shortness of breath, temperature fluctuations, sweating, lack of appetite, and weight loss. Her insomnia is partly due to her issues with vomiting, her sleep pattern is to be awake during the night often six to eight times and then wanting to lie down a lot during the day in the dark. She describes her fatigue issues as a sense of emptiness; her body feels very heavy with a lot of pain in the shoulders and upper thoracic region. She finds it hard to concentrate without being overwhelmed and has been out of school now for over a year due to her condition.

Other associated symptoms: amenorrhea, constipation

TCM Diagnosis—Tongue and Pulse:

- Tongue: pale, purple, thin with a light gray coating
- Pulse: thin, weak, deep, slightly wiry

Significant Previous Relevant Treatment History: Has seen several specialists in different fields of medicine—psychotherapist, pediatrician, neurologist, and general practitioner.

Intervention: The Neuropuncture Migraine Rx was performed over a several month period.

Results from Neuropuncture Treatment: At the end of the treatment plan, she had no anxiety symptoms but was still actively using the qigong techniques to manage any symptoms early. She was sleeping eight to nine hours a night, her migraines had stopped apart from some headaches when she felt tired or emotional, and her vomiting had completely stopped for two months. The patient's mother is over the moon with joy as is the patient, who now wants to study Neuropuncture when she grows up. She is back at school loving life!

CASE STUDY #2
Submitted by Dr. Helen L., NJ

Patient Gender: Female
Patient Age: 53

Patient Chief Complaint and Main Symptomatology: Patient suffered from frequent severe migraine headaches, mostly on the right side of her head. Headache is accompanied by nausea. There is no aura. She is also sensitive to light, strong odor, and sound. Known triggers are alcohol, dehydration, lack of sleep, stress, and menstruation period.

History of Chief Complaint: Patient reported the migraine headaches started when she was seventeen years old. She started her menstrual period at age fifteen. Her grandmother, mother, uncle, sister, cousins, and son all suffer from migraine headaches. The migraine headaches are so bad sometimes she experiences daily migraine two weeks in a row at SUD (subjective unit of discomfort) 8–9. Her migraine headaches increase before her period every month. She receives Botox injection every three months with little help. Patient suffers from high cholesterol, allergies with allergic rhinitis, dry eyes, and endometriosis. She also has severe neck pain and lower-back pain from traumatic falls in the past. Patient has a very stressful job being the vice president of a major pharmaceutical company.

Prescription Medications: Lipitor 10 mg, Effexor 5 mg, Topamax 50 mg, Naprosyn 10 mg, Zomig, Imitrex, Rhinocort

Supplements and Herbs: None

TCM Review of Systems (10 Traditional Questions):

- Dry eyes with redness sometimes; eye pain if ocular migraine

- Sinus congestion
- Neck pain and lower-back hip pain (fell numerous times); scoliosis
- TMJ
- Night sweats
- Skin: rosacea
- Mouth: ulcer sores
- Hemorrhoids
- Menopause in 2019

TCM Diagnosis—Tongue and Pulse:

- Tongue: red, thin coat, scallop with red tip
- Pulse: rapid, wiry especially in Liv position

Significant Previous Relevant Treatment History: Botox injection every three months. Acupuncture to manage the symptoms.

Intervention: The Neuropuncture Migraine Rx was performed once a week.

Results from Neuropuncture Treatment:

This patient had been treated for migraine headaches with acupuncture for the past twelve years. Traditional TCM helped her to manage the pain, but it could not break the migraine pattern. Patient often comes in when she has migraine attacks. Since applying Neuropuncture migraine prescription once a week for four weeks, she was seeing a dramatic change in her migraine pattern. After the fourth week of Neuropuncture treatments, just four sessions, she reported her migraine headaches were reduced to a 2/10 SUD. The cluster migraine headaches were much reduced. The plan was to have her come in for a follow-up treatment once a month to manage the neck and lower back pain as well as to regulate her hormonal changes to prevent frequent migraine attacks.

References

American Headache Society. "Pathophysiology of Migraine." Retrieved March 27, 2020. https://americanheadachesociety.org/wp-content/uploads/2018/05/NAP_for_Web-Pathophysiology_of_Migraine.pdf.

Burch, R., Rizzoli, P., and Loder, E. 2018. "The Prevalence and Impact of Migraine and Severe Headache in the United States: Figures and Trends From Government Health Studies." *The Journal of Head and Face Pain* 58, no. 4: 496–505.

Goadsby, P. 2012. "Pathophysiology of migraine." *Annals of Indian Academy Neurology* Suppl 1 (August 15): S15–S22.

Johns Hopkins Medicine: Health. "How a Migraine Happens." Retrieved April 1, 2020. https://www.hopkinsmedicine.org/health/conditions-and-diseases/headache/how-a-migraine-happens.

Mayo Clinic. "Migraine: Symptoms and Causes," Mayo Clinic, Retrieved April 1, 2020. https://www.mayoclinic.org/diseases-conditions/migraine-headache/symptoms-causes/syc-20360201.

Noseda, R. and R. Burstein. 2013. "Migraine pathophysiology: anatomy of the trigeminovascular pathway and associated neurological symptoms, CSD, sensitization and modulation of pain. *Pain* 154, Suppl 1 (December). doi:10.1016, pain.2013.07.021.

Orthopedic and Pain Management: Sciatica

Overview

Sciatica refers to pain that radiates along the path of the sciatica nerve, which branches from the lower back through the hips, buttocks and down each leg. Typically, sciatica affects only one side of the body. Sciatica most commonly occurs when a herniated disk, bone spur on the spine, degenerative disk from natural wear down of the disks between the vertebrae of the spine, narrowing of the spine (spinal stenosis), spondylolisthesis, osteoarthritis, traumatic injury to the lumbar spine or sciatic nerve, tumor in the lumbar spine, piriformis syndrome, or cauda equina compresses part of the sciatic nerve. This causes inflammation pain and often some tingling pins-and-needles sensation, numbness, and weakness in the affected leg, foot, and sometimes toes. Sciatica is one of the most common types of pain. As many as 40 percent of people will get it during their life, and it becomes more frequent with aging (Mayo Clinic; Harvard Health).

Signs and Symptoms

- Moderate to severe pain in lower back, hips, and buttock and down the leg
- Numbness or weakness in the lower back, buttock, leg, or foot
- Pain that worsens with movement, or loss of movement
- Pins-and-needles sensation in the legs, toes, and feet
- Loss of bowel and bladder control (due to cauda equina)

(Mayo Clinic)

Risk Factors

- **Age:** age-related changes in the spine, such as herniated disks and bone spurs
- **Obesity:** excessive body weight increase stress on the spine
- **Occupation:** jobs requiring carrying heavy loads, twisting spine, driving long distances
- **Prolonged sitting:** sedentary lifestyle
- **Diabetes:** affects the way body uses blood sugar, increases risk of nerve damage
- **Spondylolisthesis:** a vertebra of the lower spine slips out of place
- **Traumatic injury:** car accidents, sports, falling
- **Spinal stenosis:** narrowing of spinal column
- **Scoliosis or lordosis:** abnormal spinal curvature

(Mayo Clinic)

Complications

- Without treatment, sciatica can potentially cause permanent nerve damage
- Loss of feeling in the affected leg
- Weakness in the affected leg
- Loss of bowel or bladder function

(Mayo Clinic)

Neuropathophysiology of Sciatica

The sciatic nerve is the largest nerve in humans, originating in the lower back and traveling posteriorly through the lower limb as far down as the heel of the foot. The sciatic nerve innervates a significant portion of the skin and muscles of the thigh, leg, and foot.

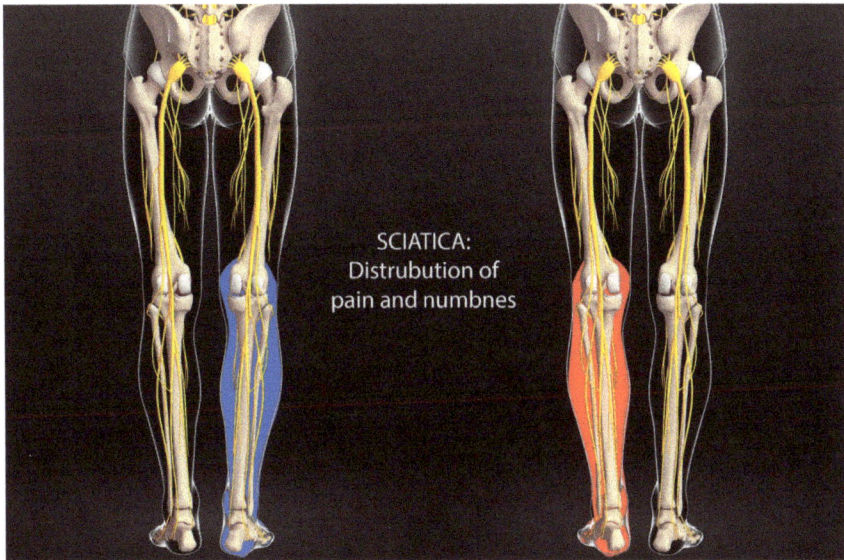

SCIATICA:
Distrubution of
pain and numbnes

fig. 2.3.1

The nerve originates from the ventral rami of spinal nerves L4 through S3 and contains fibers from both the posterior and anterior divisions of the lumbosacral plexus. After leaving the lower vertebrae, the nerve fibers converge to form a single nerve. It exits the pelvis through the greater sciatic foramen inferior to the piriformis muscle along with the pudendal nerve and vessels, inferior gluteal nerve and vessels, nerve to obturator internus, and posterior cutaneous nerve. The sciatic nerve then progresses down the posterior compartment of the thigh deep to the long head of the biceps femoris muscle, superficial to adductor magnus and short head of biceps femoris muscle, and laterally to semitendinosus and semimembranosus muscles. Just before reaching the popliteal fossa, it bifurcates into two important branches. One branch is the tibial nerve, which continues to descend in the posterior compartment of leg and foot. The other branch is the common peroneal nerve, which travels down the lateral and anterior compartment of the leg and foot (Giuffre and Jeanmonod 2020).

Normal disc   ## Herniated disc

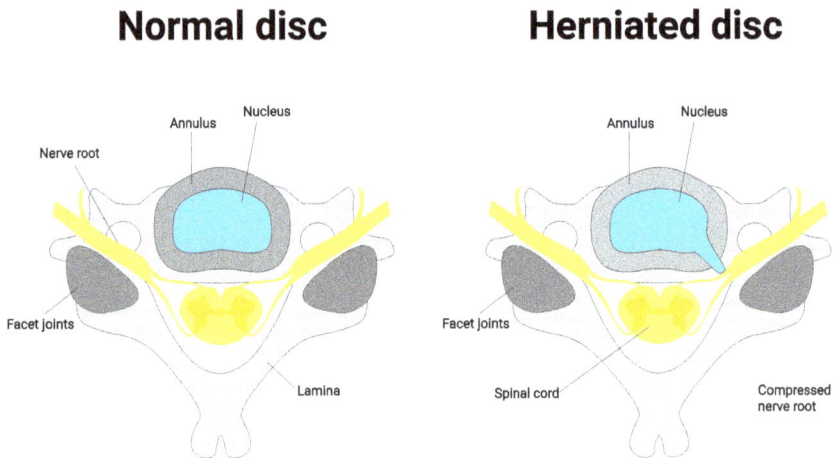

fig. 2.3.2

Neuropuncture Twenty-First-Century Medical Mindset:

Target the sciatic nerve via the lumbosacral plexus through the peroneal nerve. Reduce neural inflammation, repair the neuromuscular damage, stimulate the endogenous opioid circuit, and change the polarization of the nerve pathway for pain management and healing; target specific receptors to release beta-endorphins, enkephalins, and dynorphins for maximum pain relief; neuro-regulate and neuro-rehabilitate the sciatic nerve, common peroneal and tibial nerves, back to health.

Table II - Neuropuncture mechanisms and treatment principles

Neuropuncture neurophysiological mechanisms	Neuropuncture treatment principles
1. Local effect	1. Harness local effect
2. Spinal segmental	2. Target specific nerve
3. Endogenous Opioid Circuit (EOC)	3. Target specific neural plexus
4. Central Nervous System (CNS)	4. Target specific spinal segment
5. Neuromuscular/ Myofascial Trigger Point (MFTrP)	5. Target CNS (specific cerebral region/ release of specific neuropeptides)

Table III - Neuropuncture electrical techniques

Neuropuncture electrical techniques
1. Reduce inflammation and begin repair of soft tissue vs. strengthening soft tissues
2. Target specific receptors for specific neuropeptide release or specific cerebral region
3. Interrupt dysfunctional autonomic spinal reflexes
4. Change polarization of a specific nerve pathway
5. DCEA (Deep Cranial Electro Acupuncture Stimulation)/EAMS (Electrical Acupuncture Magnetic Stimulation)

Table 5: Neuropuncture prescription - sciatica

NEUROPUNCTURE PRESCRIPTION	
Condition	Sciatica (HNP) General Neuropuncture Rx
Neuropuncture Rx	1) HTJJ L4/5(HNP)-CPNP: EA 2) GlutMP-PMP: EA
EA Lead Placement	1) Use one lead for the affected side to connect HTJJ L4/5 to CPNP 2) Use another lead to connect 2.
Neuropuncture Dosage	EA: 25 Hz microcurrent for 25 minutes for first two treatments. Then increase to EA 2 Hz millicurrent, for 25 minutes for 2–3 x then slowing increasing up to 2-100 Hz millicurrent. You want to see the "Neuropuncture Dance" (muscle fasciculations)
Commentary	This Rx will aid in reducing neural inflammation along the affected nerves and then into the spinal segment with the HNP. The use of the millicurrent will target the EOC for pain management.

Note: The following cases had the Neuropuncture Sciatica Rx performed with varying treatment plans.

CASE STUDY #1

Submitted by Dr. Geoffrey S., FL

Patient Gender: Male

Patient Age: 47

Patient Chief Complaint and Main Symptomatology: Patient presents with sciatica pain, left leg was completely numb from waist to toes.

History of Chief Complaint: MVA — he T-boned another car and "ate" the steering wheel.

Western Medical Diagnosis: MRI confirmed a pinched nerve and compressed spine at levels S3–4.

Significant Previous Relevant Treatment History: Regular acupuncture three times previously, with some relief. Pain dropped from 8 to 4 during first three times.

Intervention: The Neuropuncture Sciatica Rx was performed.

Results from Neuropuncture Treatment:

Ten minutes into first Neuropuncture treatment time, patient felt like a "dam broke" and feeling flooded down to toes. Patient regained complete feeling and had no more pain after that single Neuropuncture treatment. Complete pain and symptom recovery.

CASE STUDY #2
Submitted by Dr. Michael C., FL

Patient Gender: Male
Patient Age: 67

Patient Chief Complaint and Main Symptomatology: Sciatica, right gluteus, leg, and foot severe pain with lower leg weakness and drop foot.

History of Chief Complaint: Patients presents with severe low-back, right gluteus maximus, hamstring, and calf pain, with accompanied right foot drop. Patient was a former professional golfer. He was at the gym, holding a kettlebell over his head, when he moved due to a distraction and felt a sharp pain and heard a "pop" in his low back and right glute. He stopped working out immediately and left the gym. The pain continued and worsened until he came to see me for an examination and treatment that same week.

Western Medical Diagnosis, Imaging, and Test:

After completing ONE (orthopedic neurological evaluation) tests and physical exam, it was determined that the patient had sciatica pain syndrome with neurological deficits in his right lower leg.

Tests completed and results:

- Straight leg at 30 degrees with pain.
- Deep tendon reflexes (DTR): right patella decreased.
- Muscle strength: Overall right-side weakness, especially right plantarflexion and dorsiflexion.
- PUP +4- bilateral PSIS, right gluteus maximus, right hamstring, right calf.
- SUD: 10/10

Significant Previous Relevant Treatment History: Over the counter (OTC) pain relievers and ice.

Intervention: The Neuropuncture Sciatica Rx was performed three times per week for two weeks.

Results from Neuropuncture Treatment:

After three Neuropuncture treatments, pain dropped from a 10/10 to a 4/10. After five treatments, pain was a 1/10 but drop foot was not responding as well as the pain and patient continued to have foot drop. It made clinical sense to the practitioner because of Neuropuncture's understanding of the pain neural mechanism and EA effects. After six sessions, two weeks, his pain was at a 0–1/10 but foot drop remained, so Neuropuncture practitioner referred patent to a colleague spine surgeon for his foot drop, and he was diagnosed after MRI confirmation of an intervertebral disc rupture that shot disc debris onto the spinal cord, inhibiting the motor spinal tracts. After an observed microdiscectomy, the patient had a 100 percent complete recovery and returned to golf. The Neuropuncture—or, for that matter, any acupuncture—would have never been able to clean the disc debris off his spinal tracts in a timely fashion and knowing that surgery was required sooner than later for a full recovery was a critical understanding.

References

Cleveland Clinic. "Sciatica." Retrieved April 2, 2020 https://my.clevelandclinic.org/health/diseases/12792-sciatica.

Giuffre, B. and R. Jeanmonod. 2020. "Anatomy, Sciatic Nerve." National Center for Biotechnology Information: Bookshelf. March 11, 2020. https://www.ncbi.nlm.nih.gov/books/NBK482431/.

Harvard Health Publishing: Harvard Medical School. "Sciatica: Of all the nerve." Retrieved April 2, 2020. https://www.health.harvard.edu/pain/sciatica-of-all-the-nerve.

Mayo Clinic. "Sciatica: Symptoms and Causes." Mayo Clinic. Retrieved April 2, 2020https://www.mayoclinic.org/diseases-conditions/sciatica/symptoms-causes/syc-20377435.

CHAPTER THREE

Internal Medicine: ENT: Loss of Smell and Taste (COVID-19)

Overview

A loss of sense of smell is known medically as anosmia; a loss of the sense of taste is known medically as ageusia. Both are increasingly being noted as symptoms of the coronavirus, COVID-19. This is not surprising, according to the American Academy of Otolaryngology–Head and Neck Surgery, which says that "viral infections are a leading cause of loss of sense of smell and taste, and COVID-19 is caused by a virus."

A variety of viruses can attack the cranial nerves related to smell and taste. COVID-19 is just one type of disease caused by a coronavirus. Coronaviruses are neuropathic. Studies showed patients with olfactory loss had six-times-higher odds of having other cranial neuropathies or family history of neurologic diseases (Stanford Medicine). Other research from UC San Diego Health suggests that if patients have smell and taste loss, they are ten times more likely to have COVID-19.

Neuropathophysiology of Loss of Smell and Taste

The olfactory nerve is the first cranial nerve and conveys special sensory information related to smell. It passes from its receptors in the nasal mucosa to the forebrain. It enters the skull through the cribriform plate of the ethmoid bone, and it then sends impulses to be interpreted at various brain regions including the temporal lobe, amygdala, and entorhinal cortex. Taste is a chemical sense. The sensory experience is produced by stimulation of specific receptors in the oral cavity. The facial nerve is the seventh cranial nerve and is responsible for taste in the anterior two thirds of the tongue. The glossopharyngeal nerve is the ninth cranial nerve; together with the vagus nerve, the tenth cranial nerve, it is responsible for taste in the posterior one third of the tongue and into the pharynx.

Taste receptors in the tongue send information to the solitary tract nucleus in the hindbrain. The nucleus projects to a specific gustatory nucleus in the thalamus and from there to the cerebral cortex. Like information for smell, taste information also goes to the limbic system (hypothalamus and amygdala). The taste receptors in the tongue have only a limited range of perception, and much of what we call taste is actually based on extra information from the olfactory system. Therefore, the sense of smell is required to judge the quality of food. During the chewing and swallowing, the odors of the food reach the olfactory nerve endings and supplement the information from the taste receptors on the tongue (Sciencedirect).

COVID-19 and other viruses are known to cause inflammation,

either directly around the nerve in the nasal lining or within the nerve itself. When the nerve is either surrounded by inflammatory molecules or has a lot of inflammation within the nerve cell body, it cannot function correctly—and that is what causes the loss or dysfunction of smell and taste (Stanford Medicine).

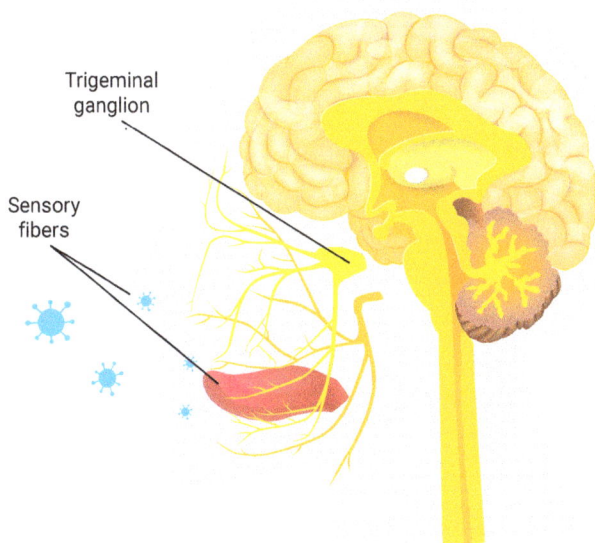

fig. 3.1.1

Neuropuncture Twenty-First-Century Medical Mindset:

Target the cranial nerves: olfactory nerve and facial, glossopharyngeal nerve via neural plexus to reduce inflammation, to unblock the sinus, neuroregulate the vagus nerve and neuro-rehabilitate the CNS back to health, to restore the sense of smell and taste.

Table II - Neuropuncture mechanisms and treatment principles

Neuropuncture neurophysiological mechanisms	Neuropuncture treatment principles
1. Local effect	1. Harness local effect
2. Spinal segmental	2. Target specific nerve
3. Endogenous Opioid Circuit (EOC)	3. Target specific neural plexus
4. Central Nervous System (CNS)	4. Target specific spinal segment
5. Neuromuscular/ Myofascial Trigger Point (MFTrP)	5. Target CNS (specific cerebral region/ release of specific neuropeptides)

Table III - Neuropuncture electrical techniques

Neuropuncture electrical techniques

1. **Reduce inflammation and begin repair of soft tissue vs. strengthening soft tissues**

2. **Target specific receptors for specific neuropeptide release or specific cerebral region**

3. Interrupt dysfunctional autonomic spinal reflexes

4. **Change polarization of a specific nerve pathway**

5. DCEA (Deep Cranial Electro Acupuncture Stimulation)/EAMS (Electrical Acupuncture Magnetic Stimulation)

Table 6: Neuropuncture prescription - loss of smell and taste

NEUROPUNCTURE PRESCRIPTION	
Condition	Loss of Sense of Smell and Taste (COVID-19)
Neuropuncture Rx	1)TriFNP-BiTong: EA(B) 2) GANP-ST6: EA(B) 3) TNP(B): EA 4) Auricular NP-CymbaConcha(B): EA
EA Lead Placement	1) Use two leads to connect TriFNP to BiTong each side bilaterally. 2) Use two leads to connect GANP to ST6 each side bilaterally 3) Use one lead to connect TNP bilaterally 4) Use one lead to connect Cymba Concha from one ear to another
Neuropuncture Dosage	Use one EA device for Rxs 1) & 2) @ 25 Hz microcurrent for 30 minutes. Can go up to 2/2–30/2-100 Hz millicurrent in upcoming treatments. Use a separate EA device on Rxs. 3) & 4) @ 2-25 Hz mixed millicurrent. Apply 2 times a week for 6 weeks.
Commentary	Targeting the CN nerves for the sense of smell, olfactory, and sense of taste, glossopharyngeal and facial, as well as supporting overall bodily stress and any neuroimmune and stress support with deep projection vagal nerve stimulation.

Note: The following case had the Neuropuncture Loss of Sense of Smell and Taste Rx performed.

CASE STUDY #1
Submitted by Dr. Helen L., NJ

Patient Gender: Female
Patient Age: 60

Patient Chief Complaint and Main Symptomatology: Complete loss of smell and taste two days after she was infected with COVID-19.

History of Chief Complaint: Patient was infected with COVID-19 on March 31, 2020. She developed a fever of 102.5 F with a sore throat and cough. She completely lost her sense of smell and taste two days after initial symptoms presented. She was sick for about one week and had a full recovery from this virus. However, it has been seven weeks, and she has not regained her sense of smell and taste. She cannot taste anything or smell her food. She has suffered chronic sinusitis and congestion most of the time for more than twenty years. She also complained of having sinus headaches and puffy eyes, especially during allergy seasons.

Western Medical Diagnosis, Imaging and Test: Patient confirmed with an antibody test that she had COVID-19.

Prescription Medications: Synthroid 0.05 mg; Xyzal for allergy; Flonase for sinus congestion.

Supplements and Herbs: Omega 3 and vitamin B complex.

TCM Review of Systems (10 Traditional Questions):

- low blood pressure
- cold hands and feet
- food sensitivities
- skin itchiness
- stomach pain
- spring allergies
- lower-back pain
- knee pain

TCM Diagnosis—Tongue and Pulse:

- Tongue: dusky, pale, and dry
- Pulse: lung pulse wiry

Significant Previous Relevant Treatment History: None

Intervention: The Neuropuncture Loss of Sense of Smell and Taste Rx was performed 2 times per week for 6 weeks total 12 treatments.

Results from Neuropuncture Treatment:

After the very first Neuropuncture treatment, the patient was tested with essential oils, with eyes closed, and she was able to identify peppermint and lemon oil by smelling them. When she returned for her follow-up treatment two days later, she reported she was able to taste vinegar in her salad at dinner and she was able to smell her shampoo the next morning when she showered. After the second treatment, again a test was done to see if smell returned; she was able to identify oregano and thyme essential oils. After the third and fourth treatments, she reported taste of food was returning but sometimes with a strange or odd taste. She reported that her sense of smell and taste returned 85–90 percent after the eighth Neuropuncture treatment. Basically, she was able to smell and taste most of the food except her favorite ice cream with chocolate mint chips. After the 12th treatment, she reported total recovery of smell and taste. Best yet, her sinuses remained opened for most of the time now. The chronic sinus congestion was much reduced. This Neuropuncture treatment for loss of sense of smell and taste due to COVID-19 demonstrated promising results for this patient and potentially others infected.

CHAPTER FOUR

Internal Medicine—Endocrine: Diabetes type 2

Overview

Type 2 diabetes is a chronic metabolic condition that affects the way the body metabolizes sugar (glucose)—an important source of fuel for the body. With type 2 diabetes, the body either resists the effects of insulin—a hormone that regulates the movement of sugar into the cells—or does not produce enough insulin to maintain normal glucose levels. Exact cause of this condition is unknown although genetics and environmental factors, such as being overweight and inactive, seem to be contributing factors. Type 2 diabetes used to be known as adult-onset diabetes, but today more children are being diagnosed with the disorder, probably due to the rise in childhood obesity (Mayo Clinic).

According to the Centers for Disease Control and Prevention July 2017 report, more than 100 million US adults are now living with diabetes or prediabetes. The report found that as of 2015, 30.3 million

Americans—9.4 percent of the US population—have diabetes. Another 84.1 million have prediabetes. People with diabetes are at increased risk of serious health complications including premature death, vision loss, heart disease, stroke, kidney failure, and amputation of toes, feet, or legs (CDC; Cleveland Clinic).

Signs and Symptoms of Diabetes

- Increased urination
- Increased hunger (especially after eating)
- Increased thirst; dry mouth
- unintended weight gain or loss
- blurred vision
- fatigue and weakness
- frequent infections; slow healing sores or cuts
- areas of darkened skin, usually in the armpits and neck
- numbness or tingling in the hands or feet
- dry and itchy skin
- frequent yeast infections or urinary tract infections

(Mayo Clinic; Cleveland Clinic)

Signs and Symptoms of Hypoglycemia (low blood sugar)

Early symptoms

- feeling weak, dizzy, hungry
- trembling and feeling shaky

- sweating
- pounding heart
- pale skin
- feeling frightened or anxious

Late symptoms

- feeling confused; cranky
- headache
- poor coordination
- bad dreams or nightmares
- unable to focus on one subject
- fainting

(Cleveland Clinic)

Risk Factors for Prediabetes and Type 2 Diabetes

- **Weight:** the fattier tissue the body has, the more resistant the cells become to insulin
- **Inactivity:** physical activity uses up glucose, makes cells more sensitive to insulin
- **Family history:** if parent or sibling has, the risk increases
- **Race:** African Americans, Hispanics, American Indians, and Asian Americans are at higher risk
- **Physical stress:** surgery or illness
- **Use of certain medications:** including steroids
- **Injury to the pancreas:** infection, tumor, surgery or accident

- **Autoimmune disease**
- **Age:** risk increases with aging due to less exercise and weight gain, same risk with children, adolescents, and younger adults
- **Gestational diabetes:** risk increases if gestational diabetes or gave birth to a baby weighing more than nine pounds.
- **Polycystic ovary syndrome:** increases risk for women
- **High blood pressure:** risk increases if high blood pressure over 140/90
- **Abnormal cholesterol and triglycerides levels:** low levels of high-density lipoprotein (HDL) and/or high triglycerides increase risk of type 2 diabetes.

(Mayo Clinic; Cleveland Clinic)

Risk Factors for Gestational Diabetes

- **Age:** women older than age 35
- **Family or personal history:** family member has type 2 diabetes or developed gestational diabetes during a previous pregnancy or delivered a very large baby or had an unexplained stillbirth.
- **Weight:** overweight before pregnancy
- **Race:** women who are black, Hispanic, American Indian, or Asian.

(Mayo Clinic)

Complications

- **Cardiovascular disease:** coronary artery disease, angina, heart attack, stroke, atherosclerosis
- **Nerve damage (neuropathy):** excess sugar can injure the walls of the tiny blood vessels, especially in the legs
- **Kidney damage (nephropathy):** can lead to kidney failure or irreversible end-stage kidney disease
- **Eye damage (retinopathy):** potentially leads to blindness, cataracts, and glaucoma
- **Foot damage:** serious infections that often heal poorly
- **Skin conditions:** more susceptible to bacterial and fungal infections
- **Hearing impairment:** more common in people with diabetes
- **Alzheimer's disease:** increased risk of dementia or Alzheimer's disease
- **Depression:** common among people with diabetes and can affect diabetes management

(Mayo Clinic)

Neuropathophysiology of Type 2 Diabetes

Type 2 diabetes is a heterogeneous disorder with varying prevalence among different ethnic groups. The pathophysiology of type 2 diabetes is characterized by peripheral insulin resistance, impaired regulation of hepatic glucose production, and declining b-cell pancreatic function, eventually leading to b-cell failure (Mahler and Adler 1999). When insulin resistance is present, the b-cell maintains normal glucose tolerance by increasing insulin output. It is only when the b-cell is incapable of releasing sufficient insulin in the presence of insulin resistance that glucose levels rise (Kahn Cooper and Del Prato 2014).

Type 2 diabetes is often accompanied by other conditions, including hypertension, high-serum low-density lipoprotein (LDL) and low-serum high-density lipoprotein (HDL). Increased free fatty acid levels, inflammatory cytokines from fat, and oxidative factors have all been implicated in the pathogenesis of metabolic syndrome (McCulloch and Robertson 2019).

Type 2 diabetes affects multiple organs and tissues in the body. Excess blood sugar decreases the elasticity of blood vessels that leads to damage of the large and small blood vessels. Renal and cardiovascular complications make type 2 diabetes one of the most morbid conditions in medicine. Modulation of the renin-angiotensin-aldosterone-system (RAAS) has been used as a protective effect for the heart and kidneys (Lambers Heerspink and Zeeuw 2011). A recent study found insulin secreted by the pancreatic b-cell plays an indispensable role in human metabolism. Biological effects of insulin are exerted by binding to insulin receptors (IRs). IRs belonging to the receptor tyrosine kinases have high affinity binding sites in the kidney proximal and distal convoluted renal tubules. This study correlates between IRs and renal sodium reabsorption and has been a major focus of researchers to understand the connection between insulin resistance and hypertension (Singh, Sharma, Kumari, and Tiwari 2019). These studies showed the importance of multiple organ involvement, respectfully being the liver, pancreas, kidneys, stomach and spleen that are strongly correlated to type 2 diabetes.

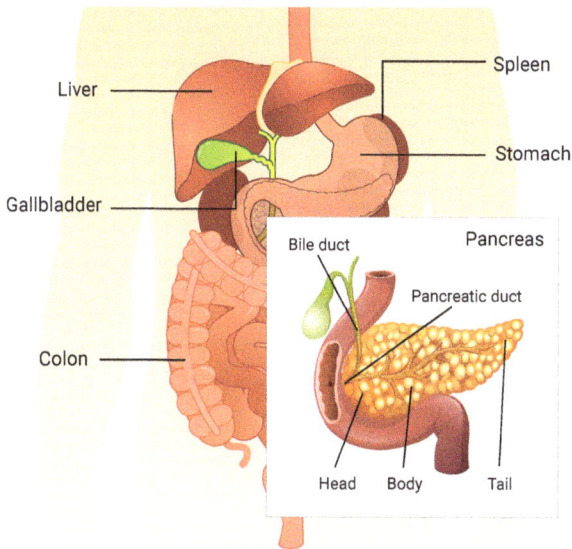

fig. 4.1.1

The central nervous system (CNS) also plays a vital role in glucose homeostasis through the control of pancreatic secretion and insulin sensitivity. One of the brain areas that is most involved in the regulation of glucose homeostasis is the hypothalamus. Four of eleven major nuclei in the hypothalamus have key roles in neuroendocrine regulations: 1) the arcuate nucleus; 2) the paraventricular nucleus; 3) the ventromedial nucleus; and 4) the lateral hypothalamic nucleus. In addition, the brainstem contains nuclei that are also implicated in the regulation of the body's energy homeostasis (Güemes and Georgiou 2018). In addition, to address the multiple organ involvement, it is crucial to include the central nervous system (CNS)—particularly the HPA axis and stress—in the treatment of type 2 diabetes.

Neuropuncture Twenty-First-Century Medical Mindset:

Target specific spinal segments to interrupt the pathological spinal visceral dysfunctional autonomic reflexes of the liver, pancreas, and kidneys; neuro-regulate the endocrine system; target the CNS and the HPA axis to neuro-rehabilitate the impaired hepatic glucose production and the declining pancreatic b-cell function.

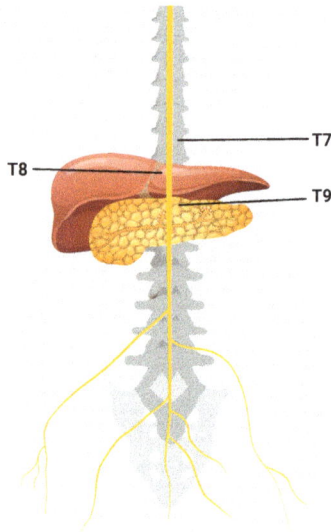

fig. 4.1.2

Table II - Neuropuncture mechanisms and treatment principles

Neuropuncture neurophysiological mechanisms	Neuropuncture treatment principles
1. Local effect	1. Harness local effect
2. Spinal segmental	2. Target specific nerve
3. Endogenous Opioid Circuit (EOC)	3. Target specific neural plexus
4. Central Nervous System (CNS)	**4. Target specific spinal segment**
5. Neuromuscular/ Myofascial Trigger Point (MFTrP)	**5. Target CNS (specific cerebral region/ release of specific neuropeptides)**

Table III - Neuropuncture electrical techniques

Neuropuncture electrical techniques
1. Reduce inflammation and begin repair of soft tissue vs. strengthening soft tissues
2. Target specific receptors for specific neuropeptide release or specific cerebral region
3. Interrupt dysfunctional autonomic spinal reflexes
4. Change polarization of a specific nerve pathway
5. DCEA (Deep Cranial Electro Acupuncture Stimulation)/EAMS (Electrical Acupuncture Magnetic Stimulation)

Table 7: Neuropuncture prescription - diabetes

NEUROPUNCTURE PRESCRIPTION	
Condition	Diabetes mellitus type 2
Neuropuncture Rx	1) Paraspinal NP level at T7–T10(B): EA 2) Paraspinal NP level with T12-L2(B): EA 3) TNP(B): EA
EA Lead Placement	1) Attach the 2-3 thoracic Paraspinal NP together with one lead and then clip 2) T12/L1/L2 Paraspinal NP. Stay on the same side of the spine for this upper portion of the protocol.
Neuropuncture Dosage	EA: 2 Hz millicurrent for 30 minutes. Apply 2 times a week for 6 weeks. You want to see the Neuropuncture Dance (muscle fasciculations).
Commentary	Targeting spinal segments of T7, T8, T9, T10, T12, L1, L2 (Liver, kidney, pancreas, stomach, and spleen function). The TNP (tibial Neuropuncture point): neuroendocrine support via pituitary activation. HPA axis regulation

Note: The following cases had the Neuropuncture Diabetic Type 2 Rx performed.

CASE STUDY #1
Submitted by Jerrie Lynn N., MT

Patient Gender: Male

Patient Age: 74

Patient Chief Complaint and Main Symptomatology: Numbness in feet, great toe feels constantly "jammed," weakness in legs, and joint pain in knees

History of Chief Complaint: Type 2 diabetes since 1995

Prescription Medications:

- Levemir injections: 24 units a.m. and 32 units at night
- metformin, 1000 mg tablets BID
- lisinopril, 40 mg, one per day
- ranitidine, 150 mg, 1 BID

Supplements and Herbs:

- Metabolic Detox Complete 1.5 scoops per day (16 gm protein) from Metabolic Maintenance
- Nordic Naturals fish oil Pro DHA with 1000 mg DHA and 700 mg EPA
- Natural vitamin E with mixed tocopherols, 400 IU

- CoQ10 200 mg, daily
- Free and Easy Wanderer herbal supplement, 5 BID

TCM Review of Systems (10 Traditional Questions):

Feels cool, chills easily. Knee and ankle pain come and go, subjective scale of pain 4–5/10, ankle pain only occasional; great toe feels heavy and numb. PUP between 2 and 3 for knees and toes. Appetite good, BM normal, slight frequency of urine, bouts of diarrhea.

TCM Diagnosis—Tongue and Pulse:

- Tongue: Moist slightly red, slightly thick with slight scallops on edges
- Pulse: Guan on right side: Spleen/stomach, soft and slightly slippery; Guan on left side: liver, wiry, kidney yin is thin

Significant Previous Relevant Treatment History:

Has received acupuncture treatment off and on for knee pain and peripheral neuropathy over the last two years.

Intervention: The Neuropuncture Diabetic Type 2 Rx was performed.

Results from Neuropuncture Treatment:

This patient has improved considerably over the past two years.

Initially, he could not even walk one block without stopping to rest due to his peripheral neuropathy and pain in his knees. Dr. Corradino gave me prescriptions that have helped the knees a lot, and the neuropathy, though improved, has not resolved completely. He can now feel all his toes and walk one mile, there is still some pain, especially in the great toe, bilaterally. Although his fasting glucose has improved, his symptoms are definitely aggravated if he indulges in carbohydrates or comes under excessive stress. Patient expressed he felt overall much improved.

CASE STUDY #2

Submitted by Dr. Michael C., FL

Patient Gender: Male
Patient Age: 52

Patient Chief Complaint and Main Symptomatology: Recently diagnosed with diabetes type 2, hypertension, and hyperlipidemia.

History of Chief Complaint:

Recently diagnosed with diabetes type 2, hypertension, and hyperlipidemia. A1C 7.2, triglycerides=174, BP=160/110. Patient was placed on three prescription medications (statin, beta blocker, metformin). I told him to give me six weeks.

Supplements and Herbs: 28-day Metabolic Detoxification

TCM Review of Systems (10 Traditional Questions): Nothing significant, all systems normal.

TCM Diagnosis—Tongue and Pulse:

- Tongue: Swollen, dry
- Pulse: slippery

Significant Previous Relevant Treatment History: MD prescribed three medications (statin, beta blocker, metformin).

Intervention: Neuropuncture treatment prescription with modification.

Practitioner treated him two times per week while utilizing two separate Neuropuncture Treatment Rxs on different days. Practitioner performed the Neuropuncture Hypertension Rx on Monday and performed the Neuropuncture Diabetic Type 2 Rx on Friday. (Neuropuncture Hypertension Rx will be explained in Volume 2.)

Results from Neuropuncture Treatment:

After 6 weeks, a total of twelve Neuropuncture treatments, this patient completely reversed all three of his conditions. His A1C went from 7.2 to 5.7, blood pressure from 160/110 to 135/80, and triglycerides from 174 to 90. Patient's prescribing physician was able to remove all his prescription medications except his statin for disease prevention.

CASE STUDY #2
Submitted by Dr. Antoinette D., CA

Patient Gender: Male
Patient Age: 49

Patient Chief Complaint and Main Symptomatology: Diabetes and high blood glucose.

History of Chief Complaint: Patient's chief complaint is diabetes type 2 mellitus. He states he is experiencing weight loss, constant thirst, dry mouth, and frequent urge to urinate. Patient reports condition improves with a low carb/sugar diet and diabetes medications. He cites aggravated condition with consumption of carbs, sugars, gluten, and yeast. He states he implemented an exercise regimen and diabetic medications. Patient indicated he wishes to reduce or eliminate medications. His profession requires him to wine and dine clients, so alcohol and eating out are frequent when traveling approx. 70 percent of the time.

Significant Previous Relevant Treatment History:

- Metformin 1,000 mg twice a day for diabetes to improve

insulin sensitivity
- Amaryl 4 mg once per day or as needed to lower blood sugar
- Zestril 2.5 mg once per day to lower blood pressure
- Lipitor 80 mg once per day for hyperlipidemia
- Actos 30 mg once per day to increase the body's sensitivity to insulin
- This is for patients whose diabetes is not sufficiently controlled with metformin alone

Supplements and Herbs: Men's One multivitamin, Prostate Plus, Propecia

TCM Review of Systems (10 Traditional Questions):

- Sleep: gets up once to go to the restroom, wakes up feeling rested
- Appetite/Thirst: WNL/thirsty
- Digestion: increased appetite
- BM/Urine: WNL/frequent urination
- Sweat/Temp: WNL/gets hot easily
- HEENT: WNL
- Pain: mild right shoulder pain
- Energy: 10/10 (10=high)
- Emotions: good

TCM Diagnosis—Tongue and Pulse:

- Tongue: pink, central crack from center almost to tip, dry, scalloped, with little coat
- Pulse: Moderate

Significant Previous Relevant Treatment History: Patient has seen his PCP for medication.

Intervention: The Neuropuncture Diabetic Type 2 Rx was performed as well as the Neuropuncture Insomnia Rx.

Results from Neuropuncture Treatment Plan:

Week 1: Improved sleep the night of the Insomnia Neuropuncture Rx, fell asleep easily, woke once for the restroom, and woke feeling rested.

Week 2: Blood glucose began to drop.

Week 3: Lower blood glucose, improved vision, gained five pounds of muscle mass, is exercising routinely, and is feeling very good overall. Blood glucose levels dropped to 144 (decreased 116 points from beginning level of 260). He does have glasses for distance vision with no change, but reports overall vision improved. Patient states he used to have "fuzzy or foggy" vision throughout the day, especially in the morning, and that he would use glasses to see the TV. He reported his vision improved, and he does not need to use glasses to see the TV now; everything looks clearer.

References

Center for Disease Control. 2020. "Diabetes." Updated May 30, 2020. https://www.cdc.gov/diabetes/basics/type2.html.

Cleveland Clinic. "Diabetes Mellitus: An Overview." Cleveland Clinic. Retrieved April 11, 2020. https://my.clevelandclinic.org/health/diseases/7104-diabetes-mellitus-an-overview.

Güemes, A. and Georgiou, P. (2018). "Review of the role of the nervous system in glucose homeostasis and future perspectives towards the management of diabetes." *Bioelectronic Medicine*. 4:9.

Johns Hopkins Medicine. "Health: Facts About Diabetes." Retrieved April 11, 2020, https://www.hopkinsmedicine.org/health/conditions-and-diseases/diabetes.

Kahn, S., Cooper, M. and S. Del Prato. (2014). Pathophysiology and Treatment of Type 2 Diabetes: Perspectives on the Past, Present and Future. *Lancet* 383(9922): 1068–1083.

Lambers Heerspink, H. and Zeeuw, D. 2011. "The Kidney in Type 2 Diabetes Therapy." *The Review of Diabetic Studies* 8, no. 3. doi: 10.1900/RDS.2011.8.392.

Mahler, R. & Adler, M. 1999." Clinical Review 2: Type 2 Diabetes Mellitus: Update on Diagnosis, Pathophysiology, and Treatment." *The Journal of Clinical Endocrinology & Metabolism* 84, no. 4 (April):

1165–71. doi: 10.1210/jcem.84.4.5612.

Mayo Clinic. 2018. "Diabetes: Symptoms and Causes." Updated April 8, 2018. https://www.mayoclinic.org/diseases-conditions/diabetes/symptoms-causes/syc-20371444.

McCulloch, D. and R. Robertson. 2019. "Pathogenesis of type 2 diabetes mellitus." *UpToDate*. October 10, 2019.

NIH: National Institute of Diabetes and Digestive and Kidney Issues. "Diabetes." Retrieved April 11, 2020. https://www.niddk.nih.gov/health-information/diabetes.

Singh, S., Sharma, R., M. Kumari, M. and S. Tiwari. 2019. "Insulin receptors in the kidneys in health and disease." *World Journal of Nephrology* 8, no. 1 (January 21, 2019):11–22.

CHAPTER 5
INTERNAL MEDICINE—BRAIN CONDITIONS: INSOMNIA

Overview

We sleep one third of our life. Humans require between seven to nine hours of quality sleep, and currently the average human sleeps six to seven hours. Insomnia is a common sleep disorder that can make it hard to fall asleep or hard to stay asleep or cause you to wake up too early and not be able to get back to sleep. Worldwide studies suggest that up to 50 percent of the world's population suffers from insomnia. Insomnia commonly leads to daytime sleepiness, lethargy, and a general feeling of being unwell, both mentally and physically. Mood swings, irritability, depression, and anxiety are common associated symptoms. Insomnia has also been associated with a higher risk of developing chronic diseases. Many people experience short-term (acute) insomnia, which lasts for days or weeks. Some people have long-term (chronic) insomnia that lasts for months or more. Insomnia may be the primary problem, or it may be associated with other medical conditions or medications (Mayo Clinic).

According to the National Sleep Foundation, 30 to 50 percent of American adult report that they have had symptoms of insomnia within the last twelve months, and 10 to 15 percent of adults claim to have chronic insomnia. Insomnia affects all age groups. One of the most common sleep disturbances in the older population is insomnia; as many as 50 percent of older adults complain about insomnia (National Sleep Foundation; Patel, D. 2020).

Signs and Symptoms

- Difficulty falling asleep at night
- Waking up during the night
- Waking up too early
- Not feeling well rested after a night's sleep
- Daytime tiredness or sleepiness
- Irritability, depression, or anxiety
- Difficulty paying attention, focusing on tasks, or remembering
- Increased errors or accidents
- Ongoing worries about sleep

(Mayo Clinic)

Risk Factors

- Travelers, particularly through multiple time zones
- Shift workers with frequent changes in shifts (day vs. night)
- The elderly (over sixty years old)

- Women in hormonal shifts during pregnancy, menstrual cycle, and menopause
- Adolescent or young adult students under a lot of stress
- Those with mental health disorders
- Certain medications such as corticosteroids, statins, alpha and beta blockers, SSRIs, etc.

(Mayo Clinic)

Complications

- Lower performance on the job or at school
- Slowed reaction time while driving and a higher risk of accidents
- Mental health disorders, such as depression, an anxiety disorder, or substance abuse
- Increased risk and severity of long-term diseases or conditions, such as high blood pressure and heart disease

Neuropathology of Insomnia

Researchers using a sophisticated MRI technique found abnormalities in the brain's white-matter tracts in patients with insomnia. White-matter tracts are bundles of axons, or long fibers of nerve cells, that connect one part of the brain to another. If white-matter tracts are impaired, communication between brain regions is disrupted. These impaired white-matter tracts are mainly involved in the regulation of sleep and wakefulness, cognitive function, and sensorimotor function. Studies found abnormalities in the thalamus and body corpus callosum—where the largest white-matter structure is in the brain—were associated with insomnia. The involvement of the thalamus in the pathology of insomnia is particularly critical, since the thalamus houses important constituents of the body's biological clock that controls the circadian rhythms (Desseilles et al. 2008).

A variety of neurochemical systems promote arousal via projections to the forebrain. Cortical and subcortical regions are excited by monoaminergic neurotransmitters, including norepinephrine (NE), serotonin (5-HT), and dopamine (DA) from the substantia nigra, ventral tegmental area, and ventral periaqueductal gray. Neurons of the basal forebrain (BF) promote cortical activation using acetylcholine (ACh) and g-aminobutyric acid (GABA). Neurons in the lateral-dorsal tegmental nuclei release ACh to excite neurons in the thalamus, hypothalamus, and brainstem (Espana, R. & Scammell, T. 2011). Research has also found that electroacupuncture stimulating acupoint Anmian enhances sleep by activating caudal nucleus tractus solitarius (CNTS), increasing concentrations of GABA, which enhances REM sleep (Cheng, CH 2011). CNTS is a series of sensory nuclei in the medulla oblongata that innervates parasympathetic preganglionic neurons, the hypothalamus and thalamus, which contribute to autonomic regulation.

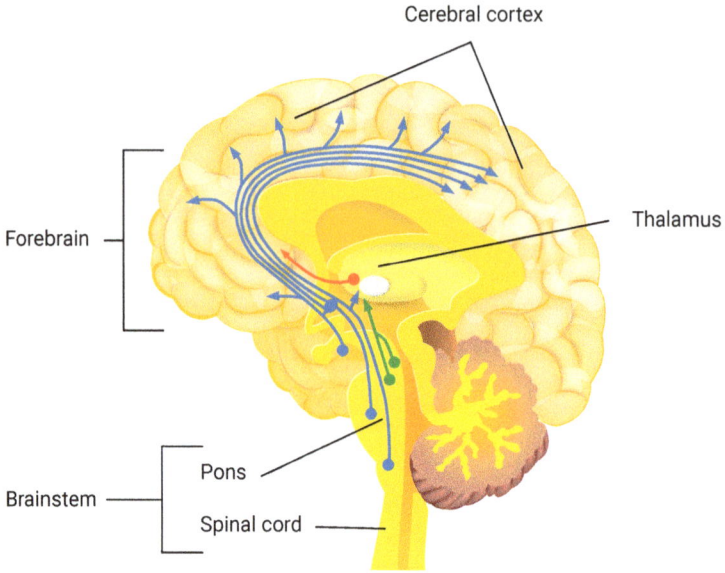

fig. 5.1.1.

Neurotransmitters and hormones play important roles in the sleep-wake cycle. GABA is responsible for shutting down or regulating neurons. Glutamine is the precursor of GABA and is thought to regulate sleep duration. Acetylcholine (ACh) neurons are very important for the initiation of REM sleep. Norepinephrine can act as both a neurotransmitter and hormone, and it is the most important with regards to the arousal from sleep. Dopamine downregulates melatonin and is responsible for waking up from sleep. Melatonin is the hormone that helps regulate circadian rhythms. The levels of melatonin are regulated by the suprachiasmatic nucleus (SCN) of the hypothalamus, which reacts to the amount of light in the environment. Serotonin helps to maintain arousal and cortical responsiveness. Cortisol is a steroid hormone and is often released in response to stress. Cortisol is released by the adrenal gland and helps the body maintain homeostasis. Adenosine is involved in promoting sleep. The most common of the adenosine antagonists is caffeine. Depression and sleep are both closely related to circadian activity (MedicalNewsToday, Li, Y. et al. 2018).

The Reticular Activating System is an extensive group of neurons that modulates the wakefulness and sleep states of the mind. It is located in the brainstem and is regulated by the neurotransmitter GABA. It filters out sensory signals by processing and downregulating incoming neural transmissions. Damage to this system can result in abnormalities in consciousness and sleep patterns.

Reticular Activating System (RAS) determines the level of alertness

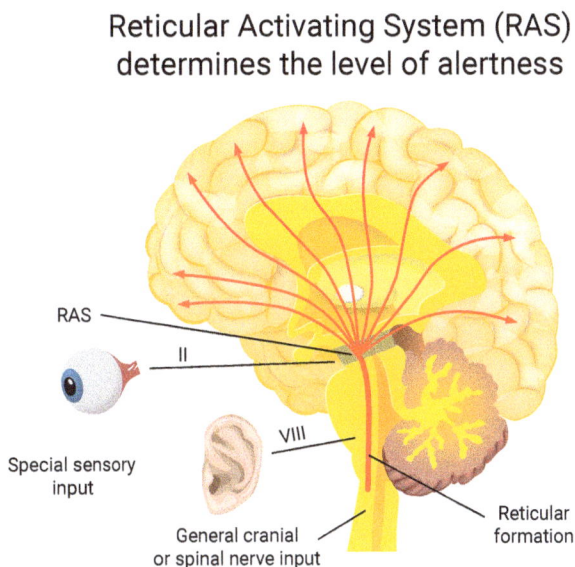

fig. 5.1.2

Sleep disturbance and daytime fatigue suggest impaired sleep-wake regulation in depressed patients. Circadian rhythm is a master clock in the brain that coordinates all the biological clocks in a living thing. The master clock is a group of about 20,000 neurons that form a structure called the suprachiasmatic nucleus, or SCN. The SCN is located in a part of the brain called the hypothalamus and receives direct input from the eyes. The SCN also controls production of melatonin, a hormone that makes you sleepy. Circadian rhythms can influence sleep-wake cycles, hormone release, eating habits and digestion, body temperature, and other important bodily functions (NIH).

Circadian Rhythms

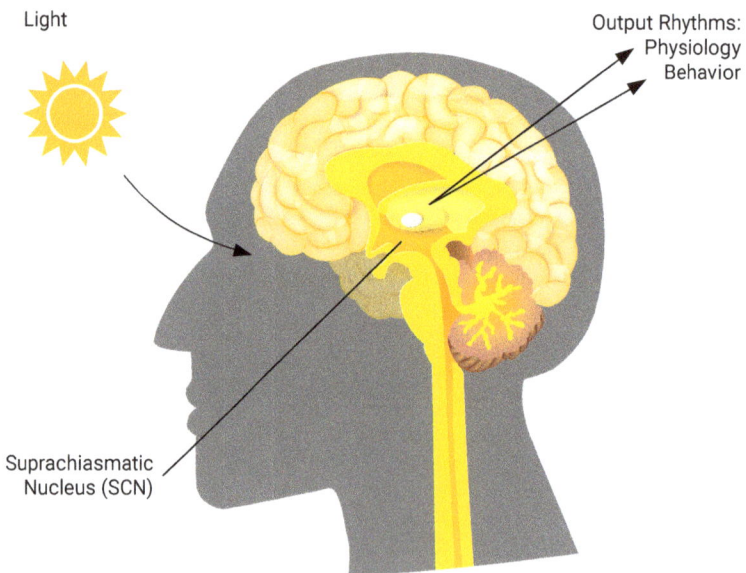

fig. 5.1.3

Neuropuncture's Twenty-First-Century Medical Mindset:

Target the central nervous system and regions of the brain in the thalamus, medulla oblongata, and, specifically, the caudal nucleus tractus solitarius to regulate sleep and wakefulness cycle. Neuro-regulate the circadian rhythms and neuro-rehabilitate the CNTS area and the brain back to normal to enhance sleep; target specific receptors to release neurochemicals GABA, benzodiazepine, and (MT1-2) melatonin, and reduce cortisol by neuro-regulating the HPA axis.

Table II - Neuropuncture mechanisms and treatment principles

Neuropuncture neurophysiological mechanisms	Neuropuncture treatment principles
1. Local effect	1. Harness local effect
2. Spinal segmental	2. Target specific nerve
3. Endogenous Opioid Circuit (EOC)	3. Target specific neural plexus
4. Central Nervous System (CNS)	4. Target specific spinal segment
5. Neuromuscular/ Myofascial Trigger Point (MFTrP)	**5. Target CNS (specific cerebral region/ release of specific neuropeptides)**

Table III - Neuropuncture electrical techniques

Neuropuncture electrical techniques

1. Reduce inflammation and begin repair of soft tissue vs. strengthening soft tissues

2. **Target specific receptors for specific neuropeptide release or specific cerebral region**

3. Interrupt dysfunctional autonomic spinal reflexes

4. Change polarization of a specific nerve pathway

5. DCEA (Deep Cranial Electro Acupuncture Stimulation)/EAMS (Electrical Acupuncture Magnetic Stimulation)

Table 8: Neuropuncture prescription - insomnia

NEUROPUNCTURE PRESCRIPTION	
Condition	Insomnia
Neuropuncture Rx	1) SiShenCong-Anmien(B): EA 2) UNP(B): EA 3) TNP(B): EA
EA Lead Placement	1) Use one lead for each side. 2) Use one lead to attach bilaterally. 3) Use one lead to connect bilaterally.
Neuropuncture Dosage	EA: 2-4 Hz millicurrent for 30 minutes. Apply 2 times per week for 4 weeks.
Commentary	This particular Neuropuncture Rx works very well for insomnia by rehabilitating the CNTS and the GABA and benzodiazepine tracts and targets the MT1-2 for melatonin support and neuroendocrine regulation of the circadian rhythm.

Note: The following cases had the Neuropuncture Insomnia Rx was performed.

CASE STUDY #1
Submitted by Jonathan W., AZ

Patient Gender: Female

Patient Age: 41

Patient Chief Complaint and Main Symptomatology: Insomnia

History of Chief Complaint:

Patient is a night-shift worker in the Emergency Department. She clumps her work schedule together so that she is often working six twelve-hour shifts in a row from seven p.m. to seven a.m., followed by eight days off. Until about two weeks ago, patient reports generally having no trouble sleeping, and she adapts to her fluctuating schedule. During her last six-day work period, she noticed she was having trouble falling asleep and staying asleep. She was woken by some noises outside and felt like when she did manage to fall asleep, the sleep was not restful. The pattern continued into her time off. Even when attempting to sleep at night, she had trouble falling and staying asleep. Patient believes she is sleeping one to two hours per night for approximately the last twelve days. Patient also reports feelings of anxiety with her job due to COVID-19.

Prescription Medications: No medications

Supplements and Herbs: Patient took Benadryl in attempt to sleep.

TCM Diagnosis—Tongue and Pulse:

- Tongue: scallops, dusky, pale, red tip, thin white coat
- Pulse: thin, deep, moderate pace

Significant Previous Relevant Treatment History: Patient took Benadryl with hopes of sleeping, but it was ineffective.

Intervention: The Neuropuncture Insomnia Rx was performed.

Results from Neuropuncture Treatment:

Ten minutes after electrical stimulation of the Neuropuncture Insomnia Rx, the practitioner checked in on the patient to find her totally asleep in the treatment room. After the treatment was over, the patient reported feeling like she had slept for an entire night and could not believe it was only 30 minutes on the table.

The following day, patient texted in to report that she went home after the treatment, had dinner, and promptly went to bed at seven p.m. Patient reports sleeping, undisturbed, until eight a.m. the following morning and felt better than she had in weeks. ☺

CASE STUDY #2

Submitted by Stephen A., Australia

Patient Gender: Female
Patient Age: 67

Patient Chief Complaint and Main Symptomatology: Chronic insomnia, difficulty losing weight

History of Chief Complaint: The problem started in 2003 (fifteen years ago). The patient goes to sleep quickly but often wakes around 11:00 p.m. or 12:00 a.m. and has great difficulty going back to sleep. She will usually get back to sleep around 3:00 or 4:00 a.m. and is waking in the morning at 7:00 a.m. Weight issues have been a problem since she was about thirteen years of age. She has been on diets her whole life, and nothing seems to work for her. Current weight is 76 kg. She is a short lady, and she feels her optimal weight would be around 55 kg.

Prescription Medications: No medications

TCM Diagnosis—Tongue and Pulse: Pulse indicated a spleen deficiency, liver excess pattern. Stomach pulse was floating and fast.

Significant Previous Relevant Treatment History: Chiropractic, naturopathic, body harmony massage. Is still seeing practitioners of these modalities; however, they have had no impact on her insomnia.

Intervention: The Neuropuncture Insomnia Rx was performed in a three-session treatment plan.

Results from Neuropuncture Treatment:

Treatment 1:

After the first treatment, patient reported that she slept better. Woke numerous times but felt she was able to get back to sleep more easily.

Treatment 2:

After second treatment, the patient reported that she had one night of good sleep and then reverted to her usual pattern.

Treatment 3:

After third treatment, the patient reported that she had slept well for three nights consecutively and is feeling like "there may be light at the end of the tunnel."

CASE STUDY #3
Submitted by Dr. Michael C., FL

Patient Gender: Female
Patient Age: 33

Patient Chief Complaint and Main Symptomatology: Insomnia and anxiety

History of Chief Complaint:

Patient presents with severe insomnia that began several years ago. Career stress and family stress have been increased since moving to the West Coast. Patient is an Iraq veteran and admits to some postwar stress.

Patient's primary care physician (PCP) has prescribed medication for both anxiety and sleep, but she is hesitant to begin medication due to fear of risk of dependency. Patient is sleeping between three and five hours per night. Restless and interrupted. No night sweats or temperature disturbances. Onset was during military deployment, and since her return, symptoms have increased.

Prescription Medications: None.

TCM Diagnosis—Tongue and Pulse:

- Tongue: red tip and edges, thick coat.
- Pulse: strong slippery

Significant Previous Relevant Treatment History: History of acupuncture and chiropractic but no major improvement.

Intervention: The Neuropuncture Insomnia Rx was performed in a nine-session treatment plan.

Results from Neuropuncture Treatment:

Patient had nine Neuropuncture sessions, and throughout the Neuropuncture treatment plan reported having a gradual increase in hours slept as well as a reduction of anxiety and reduction of feelings of overall stress. At the end of the treatment plan, patient reported a consistent six to eight hours per night of uninterrupted sleep and feeling strong in the morning and ready for the day.

References

Cheng, C. H., P. L. Yi, J. G. Lin, and F. C. Chang. 2011. "Endogenous Opiates in the Nucleus Tractus Solitarius Mediate Electroacupuncture-Induced Sleep Activities in Rats." *Evidence-Based Complementary and Alternative Medicine* 2011, Article ID 159209: 11 pages.

Desseilles, M., T. Dang-Vu, M. Schabus, V. Sterpenich, P. Maquet, and S. Schwartz. 2008. "Neuroimaging Insights into the Pathophysiology of Sleep Disorders." *Sleep* 31, no. 6.

Espana, R. and T. Scammell. 2011. "Sleep Neurobiology from a Clinical Perspective." *Sleep* 34, no. 7:845–858.

Li, Y., Y. Hao, F. Fan, and B. Zhang. 2018. "The Role of Microbiome in Insomnia, Circadian Disturbance and Depression." *Frontiers in Psychiatry* 9, article 669 (December).

Mayo Clinic. "Insomnia: Symptoms and Causes." Retrieved April 5, 2020. https://www.mayoclinic.org/diseases-conditions/insomnia/symptoms-causes/syc-20355167.

Medical News Today. "What Is Insomnia? Everything You Need to Know." Retrieved March 27, 2020. https://www.medicalnewstoday.com/articles/9155#causes.

Patel, D., J. Steinberg, and P. Patel. 2018. "Insomnia in the Elderly: A Review." *Journal of Clinical Sleep Medicine* 14, no. 6.

Internal Medicine—Brain Conditions: Parkinson's Disease

Overview

Parkinson's disease (PD) is a progressive nervous system disorder that affects movement. In general, symptoms start gradually, sometimes starting with a barely noticeable tremor in one hand. Tremors are common, but the disorder also commonly causes stiffness or slowing of movement. In early stages of PD, the arms may not swing while walking, speech may become soft or slurred, or face may show no expression. The cause of PD is unknown, but researchers found specific gene mutations or environmental toxins may play a role (Mayo Clinic). In the author's private practice, it has been his experience that there may be a connection between PD and agricultural pesticides. There has been some research of the hypothesis indicating that the pesticides enter through the nose and affect the CNI, the olfactory nerve, and thereby penetrating the brain. According to the Parkinson's Foundation, nearly one million will be living with PD in the US by 2020, which is more than the combined number of people diagnosed with multiple sclerosis, muscular dystrophy, and Lou Gehrig's disease. Approximately 60,000 Americans are diagnosed with PD each year.

Signs and Symptoms

- Decreased facial expressions
- Impaired, stooped posture and balance
- Loss of automatic movements
- Rigid muscles
- Slowed movement (bradykinesia)
- Speech changes
- Tremors
- Writing changes

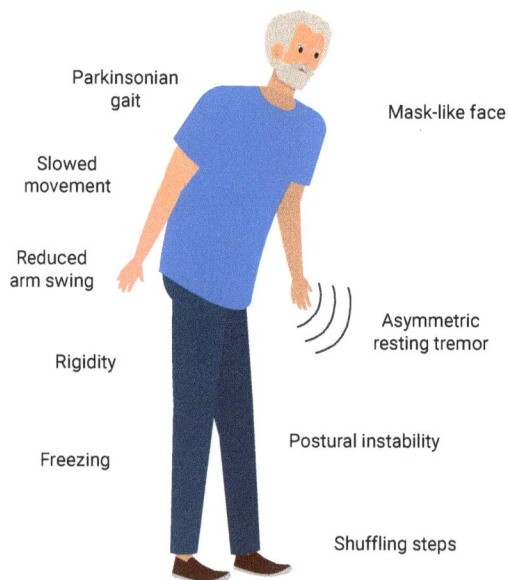

Parkinsonian gait

Slowed movement

Reduced arm swing

Rigidity

Freezing

Mask-like face

Asymmetric resting tremor

Postural instability

Shuffling steps

fig. 5.2.1

Risk Factors

- **Age:** risk increases with age, usually developing around age sixty or older. About 5 to 10 percent of people have "early onset" that begins before the age of 50.
- **Environmental factors:**
  - Area of residence: different geographic distribution
  - Head injury: traumatic brain injury
  - Occupation: certain occupational categories
- **Exposure to metals**
- **Exposure to solvents trichloroethylene (TCE) and polychlorinated biphenyls (PCBs)**
- **Exposure to toxins:** ongoing exposure to herbicides and pesticides may increase risk
- **Gender:** men are more likely to develop than women
- **Genetic:** risk may increase by about 10 to 15 percent if many close relatives have PD

(Mayo Clinic; NIH; Parkinson Foundation)

Complications

- Bladder problems: unable to control urine or difficulty urination
- Blood pressure changes: orthostatic hypotension
- Chewing and eating problems: affects muscles in the mouth
- Cognitive problems and thinking difficulties
- Constipation: slow digestive tract
- Depression and emotional changes

- Fatigue and loss of energy, especially later in the day
- Pain either in specific areas or whole body
- Restless legs syndrome
- Sexual dysfunction: decreased sexual desire or performance
- Skin problems: dandruff
- Sleep disorders: waking up frequently
- Smell dysfunction: loss of sense of smell
- Swallowing problems

(Mayo Clinic; Cleveland Clinic)

Neuropathophysiology of Parkinson's Disease

Parkinson's disease (PD) is a progressive neurological disorder characterized by bradykinesia, tremor, rigidity, and postural instability (Dickson, D., 2018). It is a multisystem disorder caused by genetic and environmental factors that produce degeneration in vulnerable populations. PD affects nerve cells (neurons) in an area of the brain called the substantia nigra. These cells normally produce dopamine, a neurotransmitter that transmits signals between areas in the brain. These signals, when working normally, coordinate smooth and balanced muscle movement. This lack of dopamine occurs especially in the part of the brain called the basal ganglia. The loss of dopamine causes PD symptoms (Parkinson's Foundation). Research studies show the neurodegeneration of the nigral-striatal tract results in a loss of dopaminergic neurons in the substantia nigra, a loss of tyrosine hydroxylase containing nerve endings in the striatum, and diminished striatal dopamine production causing abnormal motor behavior (Pardridge, W. 2005). Tyrosine hydroxylase is an enzyme for dopamine synthesis, which plays an important role in the synthesis of dopamine.

People with Parkinson's also lose the nerve endings that produce norepinephrine, the main chemical messenger of the sympathetic nervous system, which controls many autonomic functions of the body, such as heart rate and blood pressure. The loss of norepinephrine might help explain why people with PD feel fatigue or have irregular blood pressure and slow digestive tract (NIH).

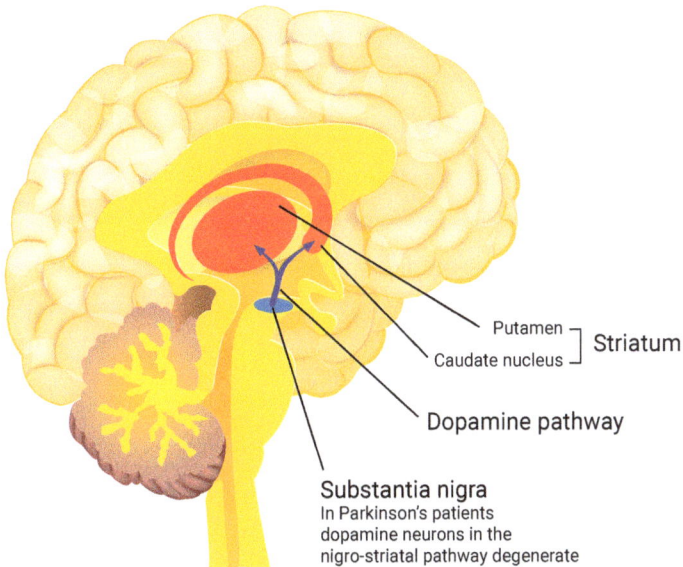

Putamen ⌐
Caudate nucleus ⌐ Striatum

Dopamine pathway

Substantia nigra
In Parkinson's patients dopamine neurons in the nigro-striatal pathway degenerate

fig. 5.2.2

Electro medicine is not a foreign idea in the treatment in PD. Deep brain stimulation (DBS) has been approved by the FDA for many neurological conditions. DBS was approved by the Food and Drug

Administration (FDA) in 1997 as a treatment for essential tremor and in April 2003 as a treatment for dystonia. The FDA approved DBS for Parkinson's disease in 2002.

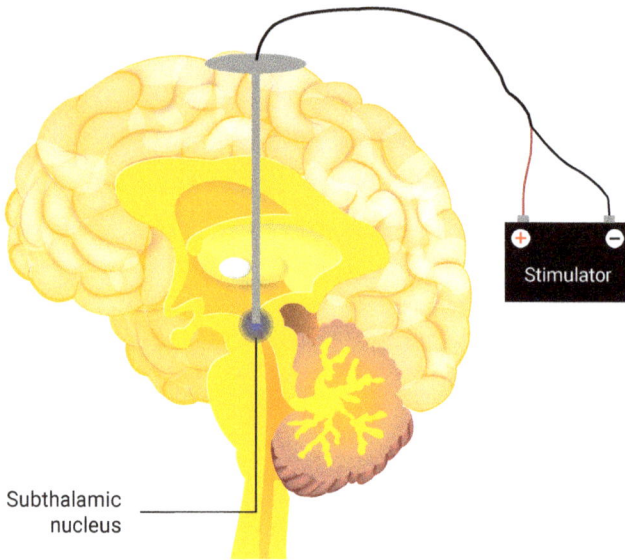

Subthalamic nucleus

fig. 5.2.3

In Parkinson's and the movement signature associated with cerebral regions.

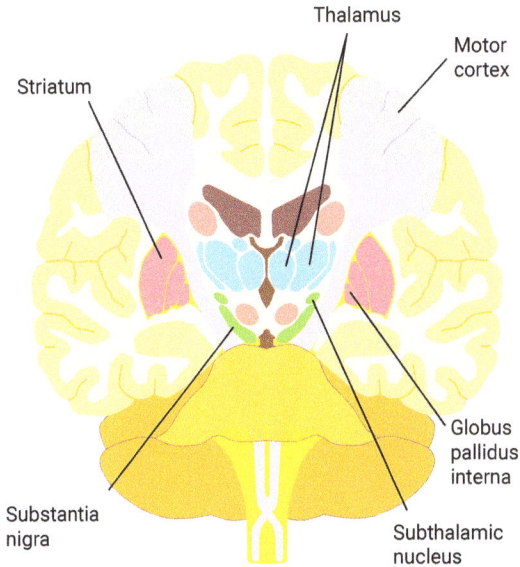

fig. 5.2.4

Neuropuncture Twenty-First-Century Medical Mindset:

Target the central nervous system and regions of the brain; neuro-rehabilitate the basal ganglia and substantia nigra and dopaminergic system. We aim to neuromodulate the dopamine neurotransmitter to ensure smooth and balanced muscle movement, target specific receptors to release specific neuropeptides, stimulate the production of tyrosine hydroxylase to improve dopamine synthesis, utilize the Neuropuncture scalp techniques to stimulate and neuro-rehabilitate the dopaminergic neurons in the substantia nigra, and produce a neuroprotective effect with the antioxidant effect of superoxide dismutase on free radicals and neuro inflammation.

Table II - Neuropuncture mechanisms and treatment principles

Neuropuncture neurophysiological mechanisms	Neuropuncture treatment principles
1. Local effect	1. Harness local effect
2. Spinal segmental	2. Target specific nerve
3. Endogenous Opioid Circuit (EOC)	3. Target specific neural plexus
4. Central Nervous System (CNS)	4. Target specific spinal segment
5. Neuromuscular/ Myofascial Trigger Point (MFTrP)	**5. Target CNS (specific cerebral region/ release of specific neuropeptides)**

Table III - Neuropuncture electrical techniques

Neuropuncture electrical techniques
1. Reduce inflammation and begin repair of soft tissue vs. strengthening soft tissues
2. Target specific receptors for specific neuropeptide release or specific cerebral region
3. Interrupt dysfunctional autonomic spinal reflexes
4. Change polarization of a specific nerve pathway
5. DCEA (Deep Cranial Electro Acupuncture Stimulation)/EAMS (Electrical Acupuncture Magnetic Stimulation)

Table 9: Neuropuncture prescription - Parkinson's disease

NEUROPUNCTURE PRESCRIPTION	
Condition	Parkinson's disease
Neuropuncture Rx	1) Du20-Du14: EA 2) DPNP-GB34(B):EA 3) St8-Sishencong(B): EA
EA Lead Placement	1) Use one lead to connect. 2) Use two leads to connect each side of the leg. 3) Use two leads to connect each side of the head.
Neuropuncture Dosage	1) EA: 100 Hz millicurrent 2) EA: 4 Hz millicurrent 3) EA: 4 Hz millicurrent Or mixed 4-100 Hz millicurrent for 30 minutes. Apply 3–5 times per week for 1–2 weeks. Then apply 2 times per week for 3 weeks.
Commentary	This Rx works very well for PD by alleviating cerebral stress and rehabilitating specific brain structures and modulating neurochemistry, increasing the production of BDNF/GDNF, dopamine, and basal ganglia and hippocampal activation, and stimulating the dopaminergic system.

Note: The following cases had the Neuropuncture Parkinson's Rx was performed.

CASE STUDY #1

Submitted by Teresa B., SC

Patient Gender: Female
Patient Age: 59

Patient Chief Complaint and Main Symptomatology: Difficulty walking: client presents stating that she is struggling to walk easily; she can take only small steps and finds it hard to walk a long distance without her legs getting very tight; sometimes she feels as if she is drunk and can't find her foot placement.

History of Chief Complaint:

Patient stated the about two months ago, she noticed a gradual onset of stiffness in her legs and back and started to feel like it was hard to walk any long distances. This progressed to the point where she has now had two falls over the last month and is struggling with balance. When she presented in clinic, she could not walk more than twenty minutes without becoming stiff and feeling fatigued. During this period, her tremor had become more pronounced, and she was struggling with fine motor skills like typing. Her anxiety intensified and ability to cope with concentration at work also became more difficult. She believes that some stressful events that happened in her personal life have led to the changes in her motor and cognitive functions.

Prescription Medications: Levodopa

TCM Diagnosis—Tongue and Pulse:

- Tongue: thin, dry, red with a tremor and no coating
- Pulse: thin, deep, weak, and rapid with a wiry quality

Significant Previous Relevant Treatment History: None

Intervention: The Neuropuncture Parkinson's Rx was performed.

Results from Neuropuncture Treatment:

After the initial several treatments, the patient found she was able to manage anxiety better. Practitioner suggested breathing exercises to further help reduce the anxiety. After the Neuropuncture treatment plan the patient is sleeping six and a half to seven hours a night. She is now able to go for a one and a half-hour walk without feeling stiffness and is no longer tripping and scuffing her feet. The strength grading on the L3/L4 and L5/S1 distribution is now a 4 out of 5. The tremor has reduced, and the patient states that she finds typing and fine motor skills easier and her cognitive abilities at work have greatly improved. The practitioner now sees her once a week for ongoing treatment to slow down the progression of the disease.

CASE STUDY #2
Submitted by Dr. Satish N., GA

Patient Gender: Male
Patient Age: 60

Patient Chief Complaint and Main Symptomatology: Patient was diagnosed with Parkinson's and presented with stooped walking, inability to turn on one foot, tremors, and speech impairment.

History of Chief Complaint: Diagnosed with Parkinson's in 2016 by his neurologist

Western Medical Diagnosis, Imaging, and Tests:

We have done his blood work and hair analysis. Hair analysis illustrated presence of aluminum and very high level of barium in his body. The blood test revealed prediabetic, thyroid antibodies; no T4 to T3 conversion, low WBC and neutrophils, extremely low vitamin D, and low levels of testosterone.

The classic test for Parkinson's which was "Fist chop flat" hand physical test was performed. He could not even do it three times properly.

Prescription Medications: Pramipexole 0.25 mg

Supplements and Herbs: No supplements yet

TCM Review of Systems (10 Traditional Questions):

- Tends to run cold
- very fatigued
- loss of appetite
- brain fogginess
- memory impairment
- balance issues

TCM Diagnosis—Tongue and Pulse:

- Pulse: fast and left guan tight and thin and thready; qi yin deficiency.
- Tongue: dry and shaking

Significant Previous Relevant Treatment History:

Treated with carbidopa and had a lot of side effects. Then switched to pramipexole 025 mg and had a lot of side effects. Patient feels very sleepy and sluggish and does not want to take pramipexole.

Intervention: The Neuropuncture Parkinson's Rx was performed.

Results from Neuropuncture Treatment:

It was amazing. After the patient's first Neuropuncture treatment, he pushed himself off the table without shaking. He got off the table and, without thinking, he started walking without any hesitation in his feet. The practitioner asked him to speak, and he started speaking, and his wife had tears in her eyes. She actually understood what he was saying without her asking him to repeat himself. He stood straighter, and his words were "I can see the ground better." Speech was much more articulated! This was our first session ever.

References

Cleveland Clinic. "Parkinson's Disease." Retrieved April 5, 2020. https://my.clevelandclinic.org/health/diseases/8525-parkinsons-disease-an-overview.

Dickson, Dennis. 2018. "Neuropathology of Parkinson Disease." *Parkinsonism and Related Disorders* 46, suppl. 1 (January):S30–S33.

Mayo Clinic. "Parkinson's Disease: Symptoms and Causes." Retrieved April 5, 2020. https://www.mayoclinic.org/diseases-conditions/parkinsons-disease/symptoms-causes/syc-20376055.

NIH: National Institute on Aging. "Parkinson's Disease." Retrieved April 5, 2020. https://www.nia.nih.gov/health/parkinsons-disease.

Pardridge, W. 2005. "Tyrosine Hydroxylase Replacement in Experimental Parkinson's Disease with Transvascular Gene Therapy." *NeuroRx: The Journal of the American Society for Experimental NeuroTherapeutics* 2, (January): 129–138.

Parkinson's Foundation. "What Is Parkinson's?" Foundation. Retrieved April 5, 2020. https://www.parkinson.org/understanding-parkinsons/what-is-parkinsons.

Internal Medicine—Brain Conditions: Restless Legs Syndrome

Overview

RLS is a condition that causes an uncontrollable urge to move the legs, usually because of an uncomfortable sensation. It typically happens in the evening or nighttime hours when sitting or lying down. Moving eases the unpleasant feeling temporarily. The feelings usually happen on both sides of the body. They can also happen on only one side, or they might start on one side and then move to the other. RLS, also known as Willis-Ekbom disease, can begin at any age and generally worsens with age. It can disrupt sleep, which interferes with daily activities. RLS affects up to 10 percent of people in the US. RLS symptoms range from mild to unbearable. They might come and go, and the intensity can vary between episodes. Symptoms almost always go away in the early morning (Mayo Clinic; NIH).

Signs and Symptoms

- Strange itching, tingling, electric, aching, pulling, or "crawling" sensation occurring deep within the legs; these sensations may also occur in the arms
- A compelling urge to move the limbs to relieve these sensations
- Restlessness, need to get up and pace, tossing and turning in bed, rubbing the legs
- Sleep disturbances and daytime sleepiness
- Involuntary, repetitive, periodic, jerking limb movements, either in sleep or while awake and at rest

Possible Risk Factors

- **Genetic:** up to 92 percent of people with RLS have a first degree relative with RLS
- **Peripheral neuropathy:** damage to the nerves
- **Chronic medical conditions:** such as Parkinson's disease, hypothyroidism, depression, fibromyalgia, diabetes, rheumatoid arthritis
- **Kidney disease:** end stage of renal disease, dialysis
- **Iron deficiency in the brain**
- **Pregnancy:** especially in the last trimester
- **Medications**: certain medications including antidepressants, allergy drugs, and anti-nausea drugs may aggravate the symptoms

(Cleveland Clinic; Hopkins Medicine)

Complications

- Difficulty falling or staying asleep
- Impairment of life quality
- Depression
- Excessive daytime drowsiness

Neuropathophysiology of Restless Leg Syndrome

RLS is a common sleep disorder related to movement characterized by an urge to move the limbs frequently, accompanied by uncomfortable and unpleasant sensations that are difficult to describe. Onset of symptoms is frequent during period of rest or inactivity. RLS has a clear circadian trend with a peak in the evening or at night that can severely compromise nocturnal sleep quality (Ferini-Stambi et al. 2018).

Studies suggest that RLS is related to a dysfunction in one of the sections of the brain that control movement (called the basal ganglia) and which uses the brain chemical dopamine. Dopamine is needed to produce smooth, purposeful muscle activity and movement. Disruption of these pathways frequently results in involuntary movements. Individuals with Parkinson's disease, another disorder of the basal ganglia's dopamine pathway, have increased chance of developing RLS (NIH). It is also known that dopamine release has a circadian fluctuation and affects the sleep/wake cycle (Ferini-Stambi, et al. 2018).

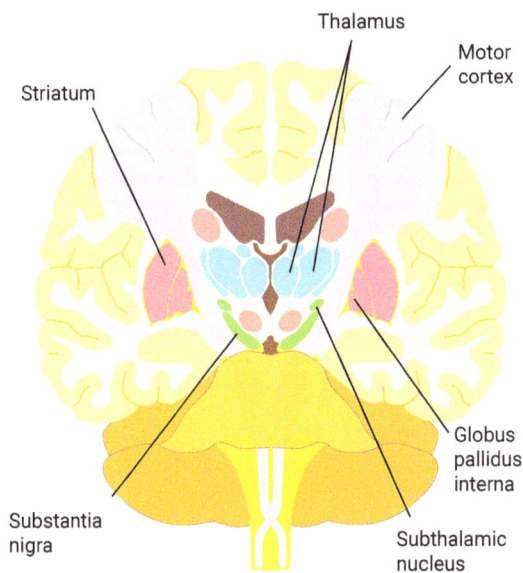

Thalamus
Motor cortex
Striatum
Globus pallidus interna
Substantia nigra
Subthalamic nucleus

fig. 5.3.1

Studies using MRI have shown decreased iron concentrations in the substantia nigra, one of the primary brain regions where dopamine-producing cells reside, consistent with iron insufficiency in the dopamine cells. Imaging studies using special radioactive chemicals have found reduced receptor and transporter function in the brain of more severely affected RLS patients (NIH, Cleveland Clinic). It was also separately reported that iron deficiency can also cause deregulation of the monoaminergic system. Inhibition of iron uptake into dopaminergic neurons not only caused mitochondrial damage, but also reduced dopamine levels and evoked abnormal activity of dopamine receptors (Matak et al. 2016).

RLS and Parkinson's disease (PD) are both common neurological disorders and have similarities. There has been much debate over whether an etiological link between these two diseases exists and whether they share a common pathophysiology. Evidence pointing toward a link includes response to dopaminergic agents in PD and RLS, suggestive of underlying dopamine dysfunction in both conditions. Studies also have shown a common pathophysiology in the role of iron in RLS and PD. While elevated iron levels in the substantia nigra contribute to oxidative stress in PD, RLS is a disorder of relative iron deficiency, with symptoms responding to replacement therapy. Despite overlapping clinical features, the mechanisms underlying RLS and PD are different (Peeraully and Tan 2012).

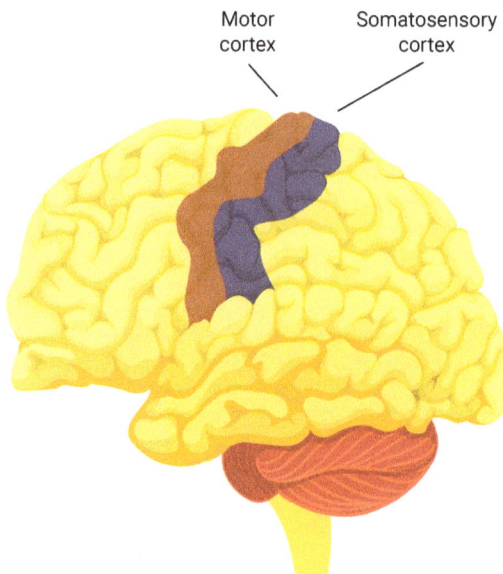

Motor cortex   Somatosensory cortex

fig. 5.3.2

Neuropuncture Twenty-First-Century Medical Mindset

Target the central nervous system and regions of the brain; neuro-rehabilitate the basal ganglia and substantia nigra to neuromodulate the dopamine and acetylcholine neurotransmitters to ensure smooth and balanced muscle movement; target specific receptors to release specific neuropeptides; stimulate CNTS for GABA and benzodiazepine and melatonin receptors to assist in sleep; utilize the Neuropuncture scalp techniques to neuro-rehabilitate the dopaminergic neurons in the substantia nigra and produce a neuroprotective effect and antioxidant effect with superoxide dismutase.

Table II - Neuropuncture mechanisms and treatment principles

Neuropuncture neurophysiological mechanisms	Neuropuncture treatment principles
1. Local effect	1. Harness local effect
2. Spinal segmental	2. Target specific nerve
3. Endogenous Opioid Circuit (EOC)	3. Target specific neural plexus
4. Central Nervous System (CNS)	4. Target specific spinal segment
5. Neuromuscular/ Myofascial Trigger Point (MFTrP)	**5. Target CNS (specific cerebral region/ release of specific neuropeptides)**

Table III - Neuropuncture electrical techniques

Neuropuncture electrical techniques

1. Reduce inflammation and begin repair of soft tissue vs. strengthening soft tissues

2. **Target specific receptors for specific neuropeptide release or specific cerebral region**

3. Interrupt dysfunctional autonomic spinal reflexes

4. Change polarization of a specific nerve pathway

5. DCEA (Deep Cranial Electro Acupuncture Stimulation)/EAMS (Electrical Acupuncture Magnetic Stimulation)

Table 10: Neuropuncture prescription - restless leg syndrome

NEUROPUNCTURE PRESCRIPTION	
Condition	Restless Leg Syndrome Rx
Neuropuncture Rx	1) Du20-Du14:EA 2) Sishencong-Anmien(B): EA 3) TNP(B):EA 4) UNP(B): EA
EA Lead Placement	1) Use one lead to connect. 2) Use two leads to connect to each side. 3) Use one lead to connect bilaterally. 4) Use one lead to connect bilaterally
Neuropuncture Dosage	EA: 100 Hz millicurrent on 1), while another Pantheon 2–4 Hz millicurrent on 2) & 3) & 4), for 30 minutes. Apply 3–5 times per week for 2 weeks. Then 2 times for 3 weeks.
Commentary	I have seen this particular Rx work very well for RLS and alleviating cerebral stress, reducing RLS symptomatology. It targets BDNF/GDNF, ACH, dopamine, GABA, plus basal ganglia activation. All included in the ROOT of RLS neuropathology. There are several Rxs so you can modify the Neuropuncture treatment plan according to your patient's needs.

Note: The following cases had the Neuropuncture RLS Rx was performed.

CASE STUDY #1
Submitted by Dr. Helen L., NJ

Patient Gender: Female
Patient Age: 88

Patient Chief Complaint and Main Symptomatology: Patient reported both her legs have terrible jerky pain, especially at night lying in bed; she sleeps only two hours at night.

History of Chief Complaint:

Patient complained having terrible jerky pain especially at night lying down. This condition has been going on for the past fifteen years, but in the past year, the pain intensity has increased. She felt intense jerky jumping pain all night. She could not sleep most of the night. There was no injury or trauma that caused this pain.

TCM Diagnosis—Tongue and Pulse:

- Tongue: thin coat with red tip
- Pulse: Heart pulse is weak and deep

Significant Previous Relevant Treatment History: None

Intervention: The Neuropuncture RLS Rx was performed.

Results from Neuropuncture Treatment:

The patient responded amazingly well. She reported after the initial Neuropuncture treatment that she went home in the afternoon and fell asleep for two hours with no pain in her legs. The same night she slept through the entire night, and there was no pain in the legs nor jumping or jerky motion. The practitioner saw her two more times with the same Neuropuncture prescription and asked her to come in after two weeks and then after one month to follow up. The practitioner has seen her once a month for three more months. Amazingly, her RLS never returned since her Neuropuncture treatments.

CASE STUDY #1
Submitted by Teresa B., SC

Patient Gender: Male
Patient Age: 63

Patient Chief Complaint and Main Symptomatology: Note this was one of the practitioner's first applications of Neuropuncture back in 2015. Patient presents with full-body restless legs since childhood, affects arms and legs. Must move all the time; cannot sleep for more than an hour. RLS causes an uncontrollable urge to move legs and arms, usually because of an uncomfortable sensation. It typically happens in the evening or nighttime hours when sitting or lying down. Moving temporarily eases the unpleasant feeling.

History of Chief Complaint:

As a child, patient remembers being told he was restless, fidgety, always squirming. During his life, he was always a busy owner of several businesses, mainly construction work. His symptoms were overlooked or deemed just "the way I am." About ten years ago, he was diagnosed with RLS after sleep study. Two years ago, a new doctor started him on Neupro Patch. He was initially getting some relief; currently he is using three patches to get any effect. His doctors have told him that he has reached maximum benefit from the patch and there is nothing else they can do and are no longer willing to prescribe it. His sister encouraged him to try something else. Patient was desperate and drove three hours to the practitioner's office.

Prescription Medications: Neupro rotigotine transdermal patch 3 mg, currently using three to get effect.

Supplements and Herbs: B complex

TCM Diagnosis–Tongue and Pulse:
- Tongue: dry and pale
- Pulse: fast and tight

Significant Previous Relevant Treatment History: None

Intervention: The Neuropuncture RLS Rx was performed.

Results from Neuropuncture Treatment:

Patient reported after the first Neuropuncture RLS treatment that he slept for three hours that evening uninterrupted. After three Neuropuncture treatments, patient reported sleeping through the night, best since childhood and maintained his new sleep pattern.

References

Cleveland Clinic. "Restless Leg Syndrome." Retrieved April 2, 2020. https://my.clevelandclinic.org/health/diseases/9497-restless-legs-syndrome.

Ferini-Stambi, L., Guilia Carli, F. Casoni, and A. Galbiati. 2018. "Restless Legs Syndrome and Parkinson Disease: A Causal Relationship Between the Two Disorders?" *Frontiers in Neurology* 9, article 991 (July).

Johns Hopkins Medicine: Neurology and Neurosurgery. "Causes of Restless Legs Syndrome." Retrieved April 2, 2020. https://www.hopkinsmedicine.org/neurology_neurosurgery/centers_clinics/restless-legs-syndrome/what-is-rls/causes.html.

Mayo Clinic. "Restless Legs Syndrome." Retrieved April 3, 2020. https://www.mayoclinic.org/diseases-conditions/restless-legs-syndrome/care-at-mayo-clinic/mac-20377180.

Matak, P,, Matak, A., Moustafa, S., Aryal, D., Benner, E., Wetsel, W., & Andrews, N. (2016). Disrupted iron homeostasis causes dopaminergic neurodegeneration in mice. *PNAS*. March, vol. 119, No. 13.

National Institute of Neurological Disorders and Stroke. "Restless Legs Syndrome Fact Sheet." Retrieved April 3, 2020. https://www.ninds.nih.gov/Disorders/Patient-Caregiver-Education/Fact-Sheets/Restless-Legs-Syndrome-Fact-Sheet.

Peeraully, T. and E. K. Tan. 2012. "Linking restless leg syndrome with Parkinson's disease: clinical, imaging and genetic evidence." *Translational Neurodegeneration* 1, no. 6.

CHAPTER 6
UROGENITAL CONDITIONS: PROSTATITIS

Overview

Prostatitis is the swelling and inflammation of the prostate gland, a walnut-size gland situated directly below the bladder in men. The prostate gland produces fluid (semen) that nourishes and transports sperm. Prostatitis often causes painful or difficult urination. Other symptoms include pain in the groin, pelvic area, or genitals and sometimes flu-like symptoms. Prostatitis affects men of all ages but tends to be more common in men age fifty or younger. This condition accounts for about two million visits to health-care providers in the US each year.

Prostatitis has a number of different etiologies. Depending on the cause, prostatitis can come on gradually or suddenly. Some types of prostatitis last for months or keep recurring (chronic prostatitis). Research has found chemicals in the urine, the immune system's response to a previous urinary tract infection, or nerve damage in the pelvic area all to be related to the cause. *(Mayo Clinic; NIH)*

Signs and Symptoms

- Pain or burning sensation when urinating (dysuria)
- Difficulty urinating, such as dribbling or hesitant urination
- Frequent urination, particularly at night (nocturia)
- Urgent need to urinate
- Cloudy urine
- Blood in the urine
- Pain in the abdomen, groin, or lower back
- Pain in the area between the scrotum and rectum (perineum)
- Pain or discomfort of the penis or testicles
- Painful ejaculation
- Flu-like signs and symptoms (with bacterial prostatitis)

Risk Factors

- Being young or middle-aged
- Having had prostatitis previously
- Having an infection in the bladder or the tube
- Having pelvic trauma, such as an injury from bicycling or horseback riding
- Using urinary catheter
- Have HIV/AIDS
- Having had a prostate biopsy

Complications

- Bacterial infection of the blood (bacteremia)
- Inflammation of the coiled tube attached to the back of the

testicle (epididymitis)

- Pus-filled cavity in the prostate (prostate abscess)
- Semen abnormalities and infertility, which can occur with chronic prostatitis

Normal prostate   **Prostatitis**

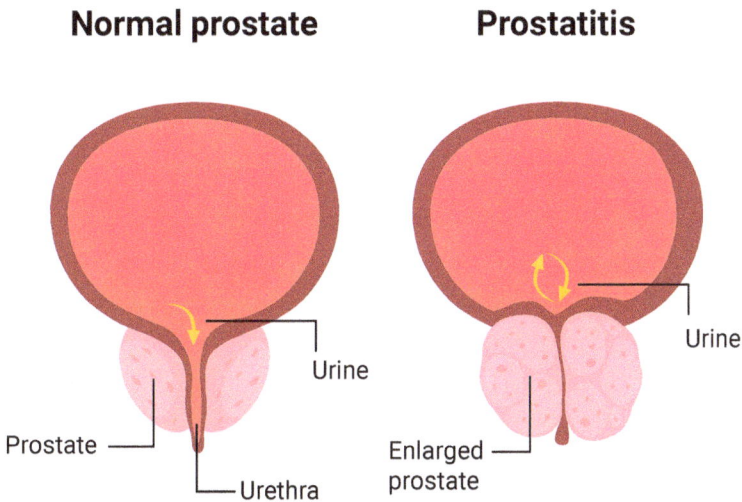

fig. 6.1.1

Neuropathophysiology of Prostatitis

The adult prostate gland grows and develops under hormonal control while its physiological functions are controlled by the autonomic nervous system. The prostate gland receives sympathetic input via the hypogastric nerve and parasympathetic input via the pelvic nerve. In addition, the hypogastric and pelvic nerves also provide sensory inputs to the gland.

The pudendal nerve (PN) originates from the sacral branches S2, S3, and S4 and carries sensation from the external genitalia and the skin of perineum and anus regions, as well as the motor supply to various pelvic muscles, including the male external urethral sphincter and the external anal sphincter. The terminal branch of the PN is the dorsal nerve of the penis. Therefore, this nerve is related to the entire pelvic area, and its compression or irritation can lead to pain.

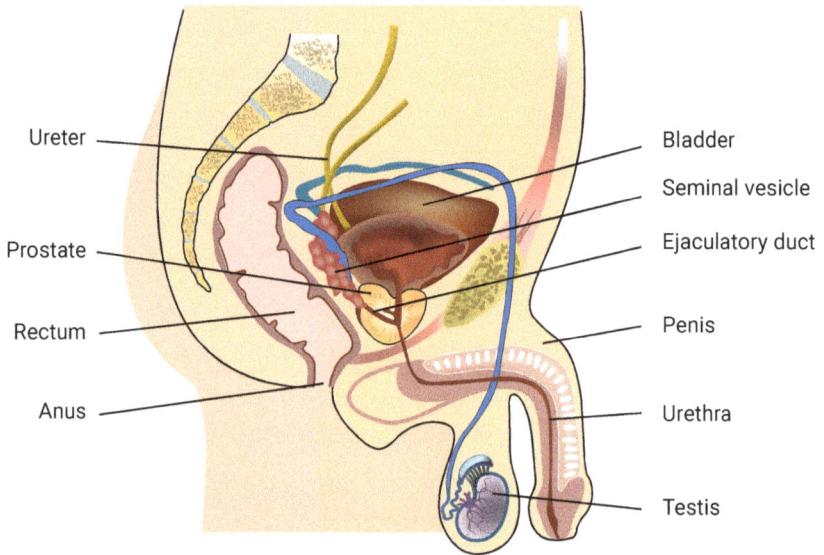

fig. 6.1.2

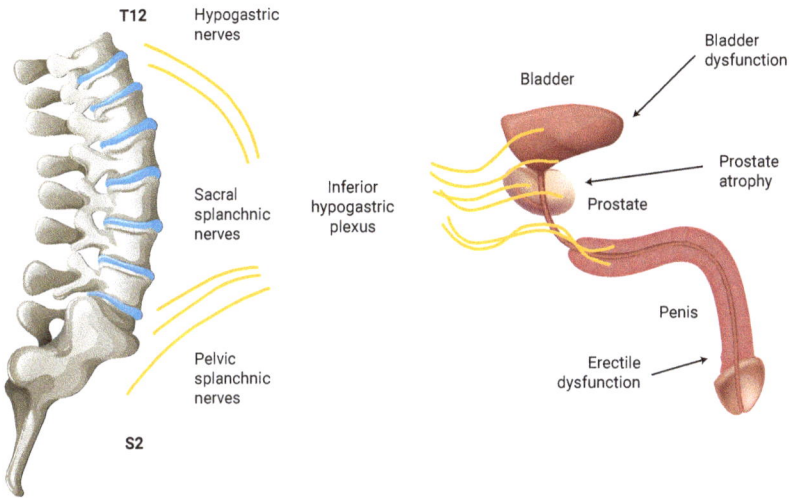

fig. 6.1.3

Neuropuncture Twenty-First-Century Medical Mindset:

Target spinal segment to interrupt dysfunctional autonomic visceral spinal reflexes of the prostate. Also target regions of the brain to neuromodulate the autonomic nervous system, neuro-regulate hormonal control via TNP, and neuro-rehabilitate the pelvic and pudendal nerve back to health while supporting neuroendocrine function.

Table II - Neuropuncture mechanisms and treatment principles

Neuropuncture neurophysiological mechanisms	Neuropuncture treatment principles
1. Local effect	1. Harness local effect
2. Spinal segmental	2. Target specific nerve
3. Endogenous Opioid Circuit (EOC)	3. Target specific neural plexus
4. Central Nervous System (CNS)	**4. Target specific spinal segment**
5. Neuromuscular/ Myofascial Trigger Point (MFTrP)	5. Target CNS (specific cerebral region/ release of specific neuropeptides)

Table III - Neuropuncture electrical techniques

Neuropuncture electrical techniques
1. Reduce inflammation and begin repair of soft tissue vs. strengthening soft tissues
2. Target specific receptors for specific neuropeptide release or specific cerebral region
3. Interrupt dysfunctional autonomic spinal reflexes
4. Change polarization of a specific nerve pathway
5. DCEA (Deep Cranial Electro Acupuncture Stimulation)/EAMS (Electrical Acupuncture Magnetic Stimulation)

Table 11: Neuropuncture prescription - prostatitis

NEUROPUNCTURE PRESCRIPTION	
Condition	Prostatitis Rx
Neuropuncture Rx	1)HTJJ T12/L2-Sacral foramen 1&2: EA 2) TNP(B):EA
EA Lead Placement	1) Use one lead to clip and attach one side of all the HTJJ (T12/L2) to (S1/S2) and then another lead to connect the same on the opposite side. 2) Then use one lead to connect the TNP(B).
Neuropuncture Dosage	First tx, begin at 2 Hz millicurrent, then move to 2–30 Hz millicurrent, all for 25–30 minutes.
Commentary	This prescription targets spinal segments of the prostate to interrupt dysfunctional autonomic spinal reflexes while having a neuroendocrine regulation effect.

Note: The following cases had the Neuropuncture Prostatitis Rx was performed.

CASE STUDY #1
Submitted by Dr. Michael C., FL

Patient Gender: Male
Patient Age: 86

Patient Chief Complaint and Main Symptomatology: Frequent urination

History of Chief Complaint:

Patient presents with nighttime frequent urination. Urinating sometimes up to ten times per night. Patient reports he awakes every hour to thirty minutes to urinate. Patient resorted to wearing adult diapers while sleeping to not continue to interrupt his sleep. Patient had a history of chronic prostatitis. This recent flare up his MD prescribed two medications without any resolve. Low-back pain is a chronic problem, but recently the pain has become so severe that he could not make it upstairs to his bed and was sleeping on the downstairs couch.

Prescription Medications: Lipitor, baby aspirin, thyroid, Flomax p.m.

Supplements and Herbs: None

TCM Diagnosis—Tongue and Pulse:

- Tongue: dry, thick coat in rear, pale edges, red dry in lung
- Pulse: choppy and full

Significant Previous Relevant Treatment History: Patient was prescribed 2 medications for his prostatitis and frequent urination.

Intervention: The Neuropuncture Prostatitis Rx was performed at a frequency of two session per week.

Results from the Neuropuncture Treatment:

Patient responded very well to the Neuropuncture treatment. He was able to handle the EA at a high intensity, voltage, without discomfort. The patient was immediately able to remove his two medication's under physical supervision and reported an instant reduction in his frequent nighttime urination. At the fourth Neuropuncture session mark, the patient's urination improved from ten times to two times, and patient reported being able to sleep up to four hours or more uninterrupted before first urination. At the completion of his Neuropuncture treatment plan the patient reported that he had no nighttime urination, he was able to remove his adult diapers, and his back pain had subsided so that he was able to return to his upstairs bed with his wife.

CASE STUDY #2
Submitted by Dr. Helen L., NJ

Patient Gender: Male
Patient Age: 39

Patient Chief Complaint and Main Symptomatology: Chronic prostatitis with painful and frequent urination; insomnia

History of Chief Complaint:

Patient complaining of pain in the lower abdominal area in March 2019; he went to his primary physician, who diagnosed as urinary tract infection (UTI) and gave him Macrobid. After taking this antibiotic, patient still had pain. He went to his urologist. He was diagnosed with chronic prostatitis. His doctor prescribed doxycycline. The antibiotics helped reduce the urinary frequency, but he was still experiencing on-and-off abdominal pain, painful urination, and urinary retention. He would wake up every night between two and four a.m., and most nights he could not go back to sleep. He came to my office in October 2019 seeking help. Patient had a history of medulloblastoma. He had brain resection on March 22, 2017, and radiation therapy (completed June 1, 2017), followed by chemotherapy. He is cancer-free now.

Prescription Medications: Doxycycline; Macrobid

Supplements and Herbs: None

TCM Review of Systems (10 Traditional Questions):

- Face: pale complexion
- Lack of energy
- Has trouble with balance, often feels light-headed
- Cold hands and feet

TCM Diagnosis—Tongue and Pulse:

- Tongue: swollen, pale, moist
- Pulse: overall weak, especially kidneys

Significant Previous Relevant Treatment History: Antibiotics

Intervention: The Neuropuncture Prostatitis Rx was performed twice a week.

Results from Neuropuncture Treatment:

He responded very well; the bladder spasm pain and urinary retention symptoms were gone completely after two Neuropuncture prostatitis Rx treatments. Insomnia was gone after one Neuropuncture insomnia Rx treatment. These treatments were done in October 2019. He reported in the recent follow-up visit that he is still sleeping through the night and no bladder symptoms now in January 2020.

CHAPTER SEVEN:
Obscure cases studies: Necrotic talus bone

CASE STUDY #1
Submitted by Dr. Michael C., FL

Patient Gender: Female
Patient Age: 13

Patient Chief Complaint and Main Symptomatology:

Patient presented with an "air boot," with sharp pain, soreness, and minor swelling. Medical doctor confirmed (L) ankle talus bone, and medial dome, avascular necrosis. Dx: Osteochondritis dissecans.

History of Chief Complaint:

Onset was two years ago. Felt popping, but no specific injury. Lots of impact, but nothing specific.

- SUD: 7–5/10, pain is off and on

- Pain medial aspect of ankle
- Medical doctor is recommending a surgery to fuse her ankle bones

Western Medical Diagnosis, Imaging, and Tests:

X-ray showed bone necrosis due to no blood flow to area. Dx: Osteochondritis dissecans: partial or complete detachment of a fragment of bone and cartilage at the joint.

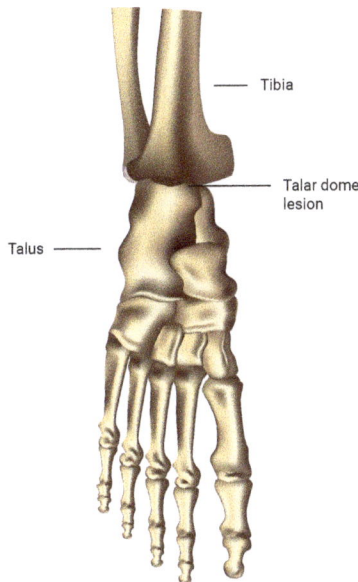

fig. 7.1.1

Neuropathophysiology of Chief Complaint

Osteochondritis dissecans is a joint condition in which bone underneath the cartilage of a joint dies due to lack of blood flow. This bone and cartilage can then break loose, causing pain and possibly hindering joint motion. This pathology occurred at the patient's (L) ankle talus bone and medial dome.

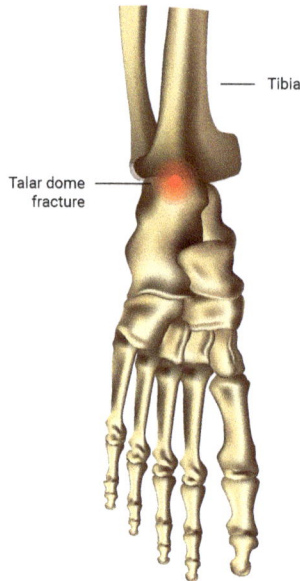

fig. 7.1.2

Prescription Medications: None

Supplements and Herbs: Supplement was prescribed during treatment: Bone Cofactors: Douglas Laboratories.

Topical homemade Chinese herbal bone liniment was applied two-three times per day.

Significant Previous Relevant Treatment History:

No specific Western treatment was performed. Patient visited orthopedist MD, who recommended an ankle fusion surgery if she does not respond to the Neuropuncture treatment.

Neuropuncture Twenty-First-Century Medical Mindset:

Target the talus bone and medial aspect of dome of tibia directly. Increase circulation and bone healing while decreasing pain and swellings. Use Neuropuncture's osteopuncture needling technique and EN (Electro-Neuropuncture) to neuromodulate the EOC and EAMS effects to heal the bone.

Table II - Neuropuncture mechanisms and treatment principles

Neuropuncture neurophysiological mechanisms	Neuropuncture treatment principles
1. Local effect	**1. Harness local effect**
2. Spinal segmental	2. Target specific nerve
3. Endogenous Opioid Circuit (EOC)	3. Target specific neural plexus
4. Central Nervous System (CNS)	4. Target specific spinal segment
5. Neuromuscular/ Myofascial Trigger Point (MFTrP)	**5. Target CNS (specific cerebral region/ release of specific neuropeptides)**

Table III - Neuropuncture electrical techniques

Neuropuncture electrical techniques

1. **Reduce inflammation and begin repair of soft tissue vs. strengthening soft tissues**

2. **Target specific receptors for specific neuropeptide release or specific cerebral region**

3. Interrupt dysfunctional autonomic spinal reflexes

4. Change polarization of a specific nerve pathway

5. **DCEA (Deep Cranial Electro Acupuncture Stimulation)/EAMS (Electrical Acupuncture Magnetic Stimulation)**

Table 12: Neuropuncture prescription - necrotic talus ankle bone

NEUROPUNCTURE PRESCRIPTION	
Condition	Necrotic talus ankle bone Rx
Neuropuncture Rx	1) GB40-Sp5: EA 2) Kid6-Bl62: EA 3) Ahsi posterior x2: EA 4) TNP-DPNP(B): EA
EA Lead Placement	1) Use one lead to clip and attach each point 1) & 2) & 3), all on the left, affected foot. This directs the current and EA stimulation directly through the necrotic bone. 4) Then use one lead to connect on the left foot as well.
Neuropuncture Dosage	First tx begin on 25 Hz microcurrent, then move to 2–30 Hz millicurrent, all for 25–30 minutes. Apply 2 treatments per week for 6 weeks.
Commentary	This prescription uses the fifth NET EAMS-electrical acupuncture magnetic stimulation effect. We also target and maximize the EOC with the dosage.

Electrical Neuropuncture Strategy:

Practitioner began with 25 Hz microcurrent to stimulate ATP

production and begin the regeneration on a cellular level. Then after two Neuropuncture sessions the EA dosage was increased to 2 Hz millicurrent in order to target and stimulate the affected bones and improve blood circulation while modulating the EOC (endogenous opioid circuit). After the fourth session the EA dosage was increased to 2–30 Hz millicurrent and applied for thirty minutes to stimulate the affected bones stronger and maximize the EOC. This mixed frequency also is implemented to target the release of endorphins for pain management and maximize the EAMS for this particular clinical case. The remaining Neuropuncture sessions remained at 2-30hz millicurrent. It was impressive to see how this young patient was able to handle the higher levels of the intensity which reached 4-5.5 on the Pantheon voltage dial.

Results from Neuropuncture Treatment:

Patient responded very well to the Neuropuncture treatment, and she was able to absorb the voltage (intensity) to 400–550 microvolts. After twelve sessions, patient returned to MD, a new X-ray was taken and clearly showed an improvement and cessation of the necrosis with an increase of blood flow. Surgery was no longer recommended. Pain was reduced to 1–2/10, no visible swellings, and +1 PUP. She was a thirteen-year-young girl, who was about to get a fusion surgery of her ankle!

Obscure Cases Studies: Descending Colon Neuropathy

CASE STUDY #1

Submitted by Dr. Michael C., FL

Patient Gender: Female

Patient Age: 16

Patient Chief Complaint and Main Symptomatology: Severe constipation with chronic bloating

History of Chief Complaint:

Onset was two years ago. Patient complained of pain and bloating in the lower abdomen accompanied by severe constipation. Her primary medical doctor took an X-ray, which concluded severe blockage. A GI specialist ran a full range of exams and labs: rectal muscles fine, no reflux, colonoscopy of ascending and descending colon all clear. The medical conclusion was poor motility of descending colon, hence the medical dx of descending neuropathy. Medical-assisted BM was necessary in that the patient had to go to the hospital and either

NEUROPUNCTURE · Case Studies and Clinical Applications Volume 1

receive a medical enema or drink a large quantity of the colonoscopy drink prep to "flush her out" every time to have BM. No BM for days, sometimes weeks.

Patient is a national equestrian. During initial medical questioning, patient reports suffering from a sciatica-like sharp pain on the left side traveling down her leg, around the onset of GI issues. Patient claims she always had been thrown or has fallen off her horses while training. She reports on-and-off low-back pain.

Western Medical Diagnosis, Imaging, and Tests:

Western medical diagnosis of "descending colon neuropathy." X-ray confirmation of severe blockage. Doctor recommended that if BM does not change, then a colostomy procedure will be the next option (the end of the large intestine is diverted through the abdominal wall, and a bag will be surgically attached for BM).

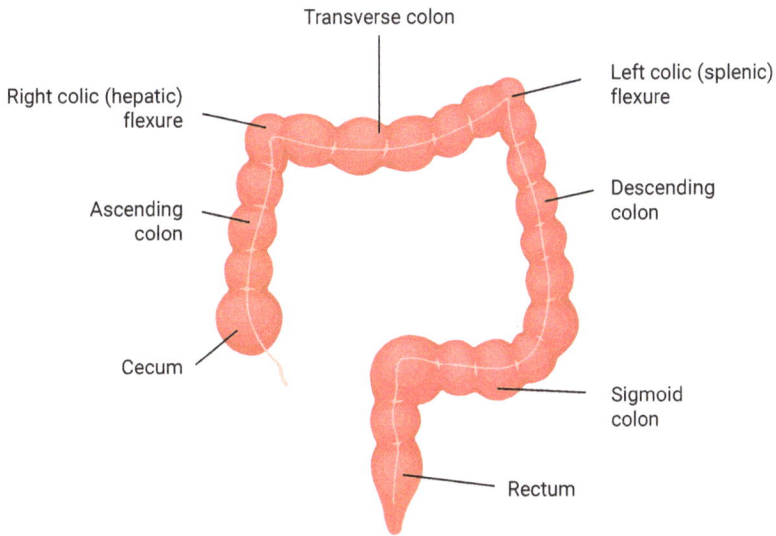

Transverse colon

Left colic (splenic) flexure

Right colic (hepatic) flexure

Descending colon

Ascending colon

Cecum

Sigmoid colon

Rectum

fig. 7.2.1

Neuropathophysiology of Chief Complaint

In this case, we look at the neurophysiology of the descending colon neuropathy, and we examine the visceral neural innervation and its spinal innervation. When we do this, we see the sacral plexus being implicated in the neural innervation to the descending colon. The patient's involvement in high-level horse riding and her history of low-back pain with shooting pain down her left leg two years ago guides the Neuropuncture investigation to the sciatic nerve, which is L4-S3. The descending colon has spinal neural innervations of S2-S4.

The pelvic splenic nerves carry parasympathetic fibers from S2-S4 spinal cord levels to the descending colon and rectum. So, we can identify that there is a crossover of neural plexuses of these two separate pathologies.

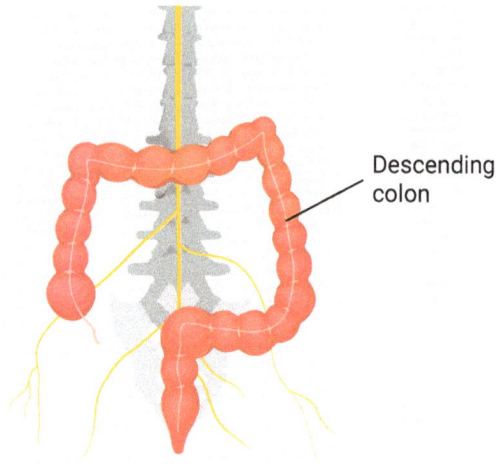

Descending colon

fig. 7.2.2

Prescription Medications: Linzess, MiraLAX, Milk of Magnesia.

Supplements and Herbs: None

TCM Review of Systems (10 Traditional Questions):

- Face: pale complexion
- Lack of energy
- Difficulty falling and staying asleep.
- Menstrual cycle two times per month, with heavy bleeding, resulting in use of NuvaRing.
- No BM for days, sometimes weeks.

- Emotionally very stressed and uncomfortable and depressed

TCM Diagnosis—Tongue and Pulse:

- Tongue: swollen, pale body, red tip, thin coat center thicker in the rear.
- Pulse: (R) moderate, slightly tight, slippery overall but not too full in SP/ST; (L) thin and weak

Significant Previous Relevant Treatment History: Has had acupuncture in the past with no results. Herbs were prescribed with no real impact. Regular routine hospital visits for medically induced bowel movements.

Neuropuncture Twenty-First-Century Medical Mindset:

Utilizing the Neuropuncture trinity, we target the lumbosacral plexus and apply the "overflow" electrophysiology theory to interrupt and regulate the dysfunctional autonomic descending colon visceral reflexes. Utilizing the "thumping" Neuropuncture "Deqi" sensation of the "Neuropuncture Dance" strongly stimulates those reflexes and surrounding muscles.

Neuromodulation and neuro-rehabilitation of the patient's lumbosacral plexus was the focus. By targeting and stimulating the peroneal and tibial nerves and their associated spinal segments, we are directing electrical stimulation into the musculovisceral spinal reflex of the descending colon.

Table II - Neuropuncture mechanisms and treatment principles

Neuropuncture neurophysiological mechanisms	Neuropuncture treatment principles
1. Local effect	1. Harness local effect
2. Spinal segmental	2. Target specific nerve
3. Endogenous Opioid Circuit (EOC)	3. Target specific neural plexus
4. Central Nervous System (CNS)	**4. Target specific spinal segment**
5. Neuromuscular/ Myofascial Trigger Point (MFTrP)	5. Target CNS (specific cerebral region/ release of specific neuropeptides)

Table III - Neuropuncture electrical techniques

Neuropuncture electrical techniques
1. Reduce inflammation and begin repair of soft tissue vs. strengthening soft tissues
2. Target specific receptors for specific neuropeptide release or specific cerebral region
3. Interrupt dysfunctional autonomic spinal reflexes
4. Change polarization of a specific nerve pathway
5. DCEA (Deep Cranial Electro Acupuncture Stimulation)/EAMS (Electrical Acupuncture Magnetic Stimulation)

Table 13: Neuropuncture prescription - descending colon neuropathy

NEUROPUNCTURE PRESCRIPTION	
Condition	Descending colon neuropathy Rx
Neuropuncture Rx	Prone tx: 1) HTJJ L5/S1-S3/PMP(L): EA 2) HTJJ L4 (B): EA 3) TNP(B): EA Supine tx: 4) Neuropuncture opioid-induced constipation Rx: ATNP-St25: EA(B)
EA Lead Placement	Use one lead to attach 1) left side only. Then use another lead to connect 2). Then use another lead to connect 3). Then on supine tx, use one lead for each side.
Neuropuncture Dosage	Prone tx: EA: 2–15 Hz millicurrent, for 25–30 minutes. Supine tx: EA: 2 Hz millicurrent, for 25–30 minutes. You want to see the "Neuropuncture Dance" (abdominal muscle fasciculations)
Commentary	The prone prescription targets spinal segments of the descending colon. The supine Neuropuncture prescription activates intestinal motility while stimulating digestive enzymes from the pancreas and liver.

Results from Neuropuncture Treatment:

Due to travel and school commitments, the practitioner was able to treat her only twice, but in twenty-four hours. On the treatment table in the first treatment, patient's intestines "rumbled," and patient felt movement and her bloating and distention immediately were reduced. Patient's emotional state of mind was instantly uplifted. After the two Neuropuncture treatments, the practitioner told the mother to text him if any changes occurred.

Mother texted the practitioner the night of the second Neuropuncture session. Patient had her first BM on her own in two years! Then the practitioner received another text from the mother the following morning. Patient had another BM that next morning and another BM one day later! So, three BM in three days, all without medical assistance after two Neuropuncture sessions.

Obscure Case Studies: Loss of Hearing

CASE STUDY #1

Submitted by Dr. Helen L., NJ

Patient Gender: Female

Patient Age: 54

Patient Chief Complaint and Main Symptomatology: Patient completely lost her hearing in her left ear since her fourth craniectomy six weeks ago.

History of Chief Complaint:

Patient reported that she had completely lost hearing in the left ear after her fourth craniectomy for resection of posterior fossa recurrent ependymoma located in the left lateral recess of the fourth ventricle. This procedure was performed six weeks ago. She was diagnosed with unilateral sensorineural hearing loss (SNHL). Patient presented with left ear hearing loss, tinnitus with low-pitch roaring noise, severe sinus congestion, and nystagmus.

The first surgery was in 1993 and third surgery in 2017, both performed in the suboccipital area; the second surgery in 2016 and fourth in 2020 were both performed on the left suboccipital area behind the left ear. She suffered from bilateral nystagmus after her second surgery. She experienced sinus congestion and tinnitus with mild decreased hearing on the left post 2016 resection. However, she found that she completely lost her hearing in her left ear after the fourth surgery.

Neuropathophysiology of Chief Complaint:

Sensory innervation to the external ear is supplied by both cranial and spinal nerves. Branches of the trigeminal, facial, and vagus nerves (CNV, VII, X) are the cranial nerve components, while the lesser occipital (C2, C3) and greater auricular (C2, C3) nerves are the spinal nerve components involved.

The vestibulocochlear nerve, also known as cranial nerve eight (CN VIII), consists of the vestibular and cochlear nerves. Each nerve has distinct nuclei within the brainstem. The vestibular nerve is primarily responsible for maintaining body balance and eye movements, while the cochlear nerve is responsible for hearing.

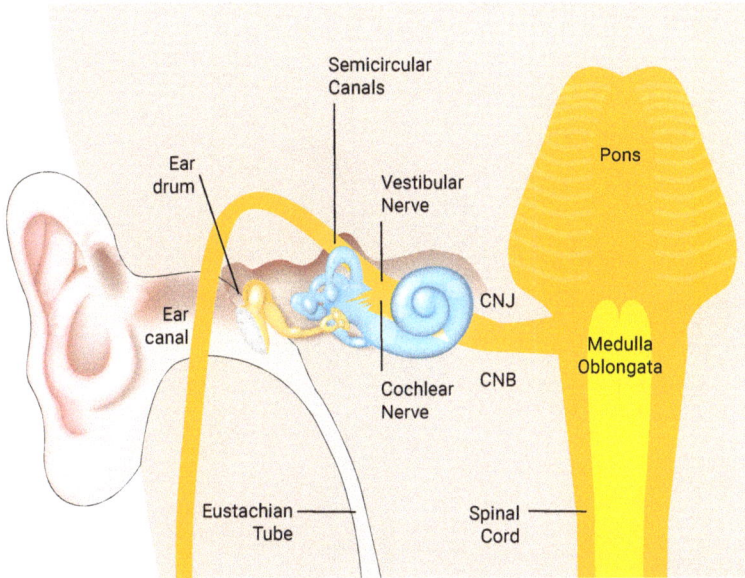

fig. 7.3.1

CN VIII injuries commonly involve the internal auditory canal or the inner ear. Symptoms such as vertigo, nystagmus, tinnitus, and sensorineural hearing loss may occur. Auditory cortex is the part of the temporal lobe that processes auditory information. The auditory pathway conveys the special sense of hearing. Information travels from the receptors in the organ of Corti of the inner ear (cochlear hair cells) to the central nervous system, carried by the vestibulocochlear nerve (CN VIII).

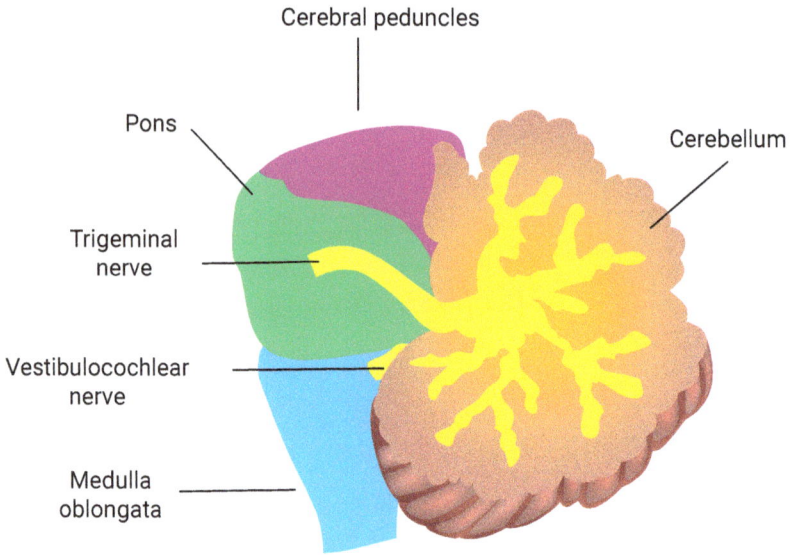

fig. 7.3.2

Prescription Medications: None.

Supplements and Herbs: None

TCM Review of Systems (10 Traditional Questions):

- insomnia or disturbed sleep
- headaches
- blurry vision
- sinusitis
- neck pain
- waking up at night to urinate
- perimenopause with hot flashes

TCM Diagnosis—Tongue and Pulse:

- Tongue: dry, slightly purple with cracks
- Pulse: slow and choppy

Significant Previous Relevant Treatment History: None.

Neuropuncture Twenty-First-Century Medical Mindset:

Reduce inflammation of the injury from the surgery to the auditory cortex. Target specific nerves CNV, VII, VIII and allow the stimulation overflow to CNX via neural plexus to rehabilitate the neurosensory pathways to the ears. Target spinal segments C2 and C3 to stimulate the vestibulocochlear nerve (CN VIII). Utilize the Neuropuncture Electrical technique #5, Deep Cranial Electrical Acupuncture Stimulation, to neuro-rehabilitate the auditory cortex and bring back the hearing.

Table II - Neuropuncture mechanisms and treatment principles

Neuropuncture neurophysiological mechanisms	Neuropuncture treatment principles
1. Local effect	1. Harness local effect
2. Spinal segmental	2. Target specific nerve
3. Endogenous Opioid Circuit (EOC)	3. Target specific neural plexus
4. Central Nervous System (CNS)	4. Target specific spinal segment
5. Neuromuscular/ Myofascial Trigger Point (MFTrP)	5. Target CNS (specific cerebral region/ release of specific neuropeptides)

Table III - Neuropuncture electrical techniques

Neuropuncture electrical techniques

1. Reduce inflammation and begin repair of soft tissue vs. strengthening soft tissues
2. Target specific receptors for specific neuropeptide release or specific cerebral region
3. Interrupt dysfunctional autonomic spinal reflexes
4. Change polarization of a specific nerve pathway
5. DCEA (Deep Cranial Electro Acupuncture Stimulation)/EAMS (Electrical Acupuncture Magnetic Stimulation)

Table 14: Neuropuncture prescription - tinnitus

NEUROPUNCTURE PRESCRIPTION	
Condition	Tinnitus (modification for Loss of Hearing) Rx
Neuropuncture Rx	1) GANP–TriFNP (Left side only) 2) HTJJ C2/C3–Auditory Cortex (bilateral)
EA Lead Placement	Use one lead for 1), left side only. Use a second lead for 2).
Neuropuncture Dosage	1) 25 Hz microcurrent for 25 minutes 2) 2 Hz millicurrent for 25 minutes, Or 2–25 mixed utilizing the appropriate current with each Rx. Apply 2x a week for 6 weeks.
Commentary	This Neuropuncture Rx targets the cranial nerves as well as the auditory cortex to rehabilitate and neuromodulate the affected nerves. The spinal segmental effect applies to the fact how the vestibulocochlear nerve innervates the upper segment of the spine before terminating in the auditory cortex.

Results from Neuropuncture Treatment:

Prior to the first Neuropuncture treatment, a quick rudimentary test to check the ability of hearing by clicking the fingernails together to make the clicking noise immediately outside of the left ear was performed. Patient reported not being able to hear anything on her left ear. Neuropuncture Tinnitus Rx was used at the first session. After completing the treatment, again using the same finger clicking test, the patient reported that she immediately able to regain some hearing. She also reported her sinus drained during the treatment. After the 2nd treatment, another rudimentary test was done to test the hearing. A sound produced from rubbing two fingers together was performed. She reported that she was able to hear the sound which is much softer than the clicking of fingernails tested previously. The sinus congestion was much reduced after 2nd treatment. After the 3rd treatment, she was able to hear conversation if spoken close to her left ear. Patient reported the low pitch roaring noises had significantly reduced to a SUD scale of 2/10. At this time, she is able to hear full conversations between family members and listening to news reporters on the television.

An audiogram test was performed after nine treatments. Patient showed improvement of her left ear that she could hear from 500 to 2000Hz, she still showed poor hearing for the low and high pitch sound, but this is certainly better than the complete loss of hearing.

FUTURE THOUGHTS

It is the authors' hope that this Volume 1 of Neuropuncture clinical case studies will help to highlight the effectiveness of the Neuropuncture system and aid in bridging the gap between acupuncture and conventional Western medicine. We have laid out many very successful clinical cases from practitioners from around the world who have properly implemented this special neuroscience acupuncture system, and we want to thank them for their commitment to our profession and their devotion to their patients' health. We hope that we have presented that Neuropuncture's techniques are neuromodulating, neuro-regulating, and neuro-rehabilitating. When we apply twenty-first-century medical sciences to our classical acupuncture model, we are liberating this very powerful medical tool from the trappings of historical language and outdated and misunderstood ancient language.

Looking into the future of Neuropuncture is to place it in the heart of mainstream Western medicine—hospital settings, operating rooms, emergency rooms, integration with addiction medicine clinics, women's health facilities, orthopedic surgical centers, internal medicine departments, and integrated pain management centers. I urge you to continue your interest and training in Neuropuncture and help us reach every corner of the world.

Volume 2 List of Conditions

Mental Health:

- Addiction (smoking, opioid)
- Bipolar Disorder

Internal Medicine—ENT:

- Bell's Palsy
- Ophthalmology
- Nystagmus
- Tinnitus
- Trigeminal neuralgia

Internal Medicine—Gastrointestinal:

- Constipation
- Dysphasia
- Gastroparesis
- Internal Medicine—Cardiology:
- Atrial Fibrillation
- Hypertension

Internal Medicine—Urogenital:

- Kidney stones
- Incontinence/neurogenic bladder

Obscure case section:

- Spinal cord injury

Volume 3—Women's Health

This volume will be devoted to women's health conditions and will cover a variety of women's health ailments yet to be announced.

For more information and Neuropuncture training, please contact the following:

https://neuropuncture.com
neuropuncture@gmail.com

A Collection of Additional Neuropuncture References

Becker, Robert, MD. *The Body Electric: Electromagnetism and the foundation of life.* New York: Quill, 1985. Print.

Bensky, Dan, and John O'Connor. *Acupuncture: A Comprehensive Text.* Seattle: Eastland Press, 1992. Print.

Corradino, Michael. *Neuropuncture: A Clinical Manual.* England: Singing Dragon, 2017. Print.

Corradino, Michael. *Neuropuncture: A Neuroscience Acupuncture System.* San Diego: AG Creative Solutions: 2012. Print.

Cummings, Mike, and Adrian White. *An Introduction to Western Medical Acupuncture.* New York: Churchill Livingstone, 2008. Print.

DeLisa, Joel A. "Rehabilitation Medicine." 3rd ed. Philadelphia: Lippincott-Raven, 1998. Print.

Department of Pain Management. *Afferent Neural Branching at Human Acupuncture Points.* Melbourne: Department of Pain Management, 2011. Print.

Filshie, Jacqueline, and Adrian White. *Medical Acupuncture: A Western Scientific Approach.* New York: Churchill Livingstone, 1998. Print.

Gray, Henry. *Gray's Anatomy: Descriptive and Surgical.* New York:

Bounty Books, 1997. Print.

Jing-Nuan, Wu. *Ling Shu or The Spiritual Pivot.* Hawaii: University of Hawaii Press, 1993. Print.

Jing-Nuan, Wu. *Ling Shu or The Spiritual Pivot.* Hawaii: University of Hawaii Press, 1993. Print.

Liangyue, Deng, and Gan Yijun. *Chinese Acupuncture and Moxibustion.* Beijing: Foreign Languages Press, 1987. Print.

Maciocia, Giovanni. *The Foundations of Chinese Medicine: A Comprehensive Text for Acupuncturists and Herbalists.* Edinburgh London Melbourne and New York: Churchill Livingstone, 1989. Print.

Marieb, Elaine N. *Human Anatomy and Physiology.* Redwood City: Benjamin-Cummings Publishing, 1992. Print.

Narahari, Joshi. "Electroacupuncture Effects on the Disintegration of Beta Amyloid Sheets: Its Application to Alzheimer's Disease." *Medical Acupuncture* 24, no. 3, 2012.

Neuroscience Research Center, Beijing Medical University. *Physiology of Acupuncture: Review of Thirty years of Research.* Beijing: Neuroscience Research Center, Beijing Medical University, 1997. Print.

Neuroscience Research Institute, Peking University. *Acupuncture:*

neuropeptide release produced by electrical stimulation of different frequencies. Peking: Neuroscience Research Institute, Peking University, 2003. Print.

Neuroscience Research Institute, Peking University. *Relations between brain network activation and analgesic effect induced by low vs. high frequency electrical acupoint stimulation in different subjects: a functional magnetic resonance imaging study.* Peking: Neuroscience Research Institute, Peking University, 2003. Print.

Susan Samueli Center for Integrative Medicine. *Point Specificity in Acupuncture.* California: Susan Samueli Center for Integrative Medicine, 2012. Print.

Wallace, Mark S. "Pain Medicine and Management." New York: McGraw Hill Medical, 2005.

Yan Jiang, MD, PhD. "Acupuncture in the treatment of Parkinson's disease." *North American Journal of Medical Science* 2, no. 1 (2009):32--34. DOI: *10.7156/najms.2009.0201*

www.ingramcontent.com/pod-product-compliance
Lightning Source LLC
Chambersburg PA
CBHW041214030426
42336CB00023B/3338